Art Schatz
D.V.M.

DR. DANGER

Life Story Of A Rural Veterinarian

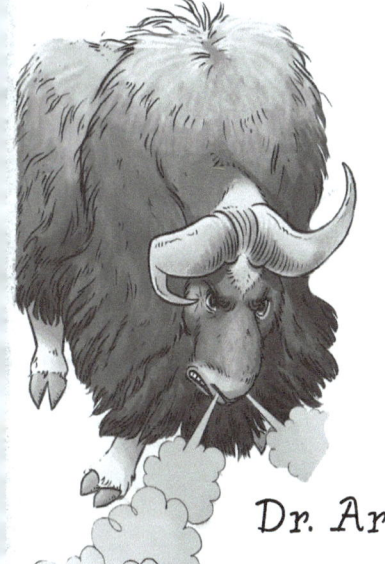

Dr. Art Schatz, DVM

◆ FriesenPress

One Printers Way
Altona, MB R0G 0B0
Canada

www.friesenpress.com

Copyright © 2025 by Dr. Art Schatz, DVM
First Edition — 2025

All rights reserved.

No part of this publication may be reproduced in any form, or by any means, electronic or mechanical, including photocopying, recording, or any information browsing, storage, or retrieval system, without permission in writing from FriesenPress.

Cover Illustration by Penny Nicoles

ISBN
978-1-03-833135-9 (Hardcover)
978-1-03-833134-2 (Paperback)
978-1-03-833136-6 (eBook)

1. BIOGRAPHY & AUTOBIOGRAPHY, MEDICAL

Distributed to the trade by The Ingram Book Company

This book is dedicated to my wife Eileen for her patience and support over 52 years of marriage and to our children Kerry Ann, Travis, Lanny and Jason Schatz. Thanks also to my sisters Evelyn Dew and Bernice Brosseau for their support over the years.

Special dedication also to my late hard working and supportive parents Mathew and Katherine Schatz as well as my late brothers Everett and Benny Schatz.

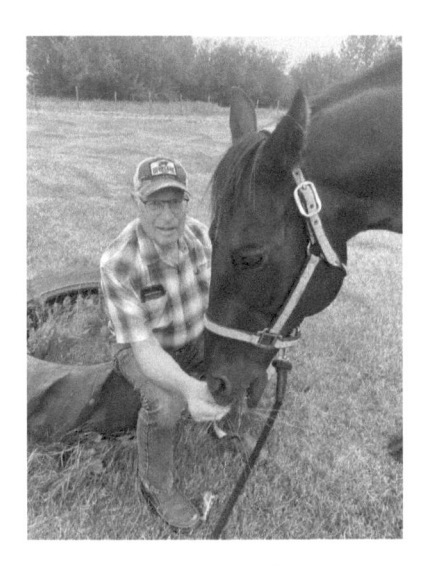

Old lame Man and Old lame Horse

To the Readers

During this book, I do mention the actual names of various people (work associates, former teachers, etc.) but when I discuss actual veterinary practice cases fictional names of the clients (owners) are used. I have tried to display no malicious intent as I relay some of the "stories". Please bear in mind that I have tried to tell my stories without too much embellishment. I apologize for any inaccuracy and also if I have failed to mention the names of some former associates and colleagues.

My hope is that my story will provide some amusement to the reader as well as some perspective about rural veterinary practice. As much as possible I have attempted to describe medical terms and conditions in layman's language. Forgive me if at times my views stray towards being a bit political; I am the result of various "knocks" in my lifetime (as well as some cow kicks to my head!).

Acknowledgements

Special thank you to Marie Coristine, work colleague and friend for typing the majority of the book.

The Wainwright area history book, *Buffalo Tales and Trails*.

Emma, Zane and the rest of the Fairview Public Library for aiding in the submission of this book to the publisher.

Dr. Phil Buote, Complaints Director, Alberta Veterinary Medical Association for advice in regards to Chapter Seventeen.

Table of Contents

Chapter One: The Formative Years for a Veterinarian	1
Chapter Two: My College Years	19
Chapter Three: Veterinary Practice: The First Half Year!	37
Chapter Four: A Tribute to Dr. Leitch	45
Chapter Five: Rabies	63
Chapter Six: Boom and Bust	69
Chapter Seven: Narcolepsy and Fatigue	73
Chapter Eight: Practice Reflections	81
Chapter Nine: Guts, Gore and More	107
Chapter Ten: Prolapses	113
Chapter Eleven: Valuable Associates	121
Chapter Twelve: Muskox: A Tale of Woe	127
Chapter Thirteen: The College Years at Fairview	135
Chapter Fourteen: More Practice Reflections	161
Chapter Fifteen: A Few Personal Notes	177
Chapter Sixteen: Westview Ranch Alias Poverty Acres	195
Chapter Seventeen: Professional Governance	205
Chapter Eighteen: Thoughts: Future of the Veterinary Profession	209

Chapter One

THE FORMATIVE YEARS FOR A VETERINARIAN

MAY 2, 1945 marked my arrival on the planet Earth. My parents Mathew (Matt) and Katherine (Katey) Schatz operated a small mixed farm located ½ mile north of the small southern Alberta town of Bow Island.

Horses, milk cows, pigs, chickens, sheep, ducks, turkeys and geese graced the farmyard along with a dog or two and numerous cats.

One of my first memories involved a large nasty black turkey tom my family called Old Gobble Gobble. If he spotted me wandering around the farmyard, he delighted in making a run for me with wings beating forward, nasty neck reaching forward so he could peck me and jumping out in front of me with his clawed legs striking at me.

Luckily, most of these occasions, one of my older sisters (Bernice and Evelyn) or one of my older brothers (Everett and

Benny) would intervene on Gobble Gobble's attacks on me by yelling at him and charging back on him (he was a coward with anyone perceived to be bigger than him)!

One day I wandered into a small building that provided shelter for the dry sows (mother pigs that were either not pregnant or pregnant, i.e. not nursing piglets). The building was long, no windows and only a small door entrance. Old Gobble Gobble must have spotted me go into the narrow building as he suddenly appeared in the doorway entrance. He had me trapped, I couldn't run away by him and he attacked me with demonic fury! I flailed my arms in front of me, screaming and crying while he pecked me, scratched me and beat me with his wings.

My brother Benny must have heard the ruckus for he appeared at the doorway; my situation amused him as he laughed and laughed. After what seemed an eternity, he relented from his mirth, gave Old Gobble Gobble a kick to his butt and picked me up to safety.

Other early memories were happier such as playing with kittens, little ducklings, baby chicks, newborn piglets and baby calves. I was a very shy boy so perhaps an affinity to animals was attributed to my shyness.

One day my Dad came home with two very young badger kits. Dad said their mother had been killed (he didn't say how?). The prairie badger dug large burrows and the badger holes were a hazard for horses and cows. If a horse or cow inadvertently stepped in a badger hole, they might suffer a broken leg. Badgers did serve a useful purpose though on the prairies as they preyed upon the Richardson ground squirrel (gopher). Gophers could cause a lot of damage to farmer's crops of wheat, barley or oats.

Benny and I bottle fed the badger kits, fed them our round steak (bologna) and tube steak (wiener) sandwiches. For the perverse reason of just being little bothersome brothers, we named them after our sisters Bernice and Evelyn.

THE FORMATIVE YEARS FOR A VETERINARIAN

I think my Dad had an ulterior motive in bringing those orphan badger kits home to us; Benny and I spent hours snaring, drowning out gophers to feed to the baby badgers. We also caught mice to feed them. I think Dad was pleased with our pest reduction program.

The badgers would respond to their names being called (or maybe to the lure of food). They were rather cuddly to begin with but by the end of summer, they started to display the innate snarly personality of badgers. It so happened that a travelling circus stopped in Bow Island and Dad sold our badgers to the circus. Benny and I were not totally heart-broken as Dad gave us a few pennies for candy. Selling to the circus would be severely condemned by animal welfare advocates of today but I am amazed at how much our society has evolved as to how people think of animal welfare.

When I was 5 years old, Dad came home one day with an orphan lamb given to him by a neighboring farmer. I named the lamb Buddy, and I was happy bottle feeding and caring for him, he followed me around the farm like a dog. However, Buddy the lamb turned into a ram as he matured. Following his natural instinct and his newly formed hormones, Buddy displayed the nastiness of charging me and head bunting me whenever he caught me unaware. I cried and yelled at him; I was very angry with him.

One day I noticed that he was gone, Dad said that he had sold him. I now cried in sorrow, in retrospect, it was a lesson in the reality of raising farm animals.

When I was 6 years old, my older brothers had made a trip to the South Saskatchewan River (about 6 miles north of our farm). There were cottonwood trees along this river, as well as saskatoon bushes. Benny and Everett found an owlet on the ground below a cottonwood tree. I now had another summer project; catching mice and gophers to feed the owlet. I called him Goofy, as summer went on he matured into a magnificent horned owl. Our barn had a large door to the hay loft, this door could be opened down so large lifts of hay could be hoisted into the loft.

Goofy learned to swoop down and land gently on one's outstretched arm. When not busy hunting for mice, Goofy would perch on the ledge of the open hay loft door.

One day, a salesman drove into our farmyard, as he got out of his car, Goofy swooped down towards him. The salesman jumped back into his car and sped away!

Goofy was gone for a month, then returned to our farm and companionship for a few days. He left again and returned after 6 months, then disappeared to never return again. I like to think that he met a mate and lived a long happy life.

Mom and Dad milked a number of dairy cows and for a number of years, Dad delivered bottles of milk and cream to residents of the town of Bow Island. Some milk was separated into cream and skim milk. One of my early childhood chores was turning the handle of the cream separator machine!

Mom made butter from the cream and another chore for me was to turn the handle of the butter churn. Mom sold the butter (other than our own use) to housewives in town.

Skim milk was a by-product of the cream separator; the skim milk was still nutritious even though devoid of most of the butter fat portion. It was fed to the pigs and to "pail bunter calves". The pail bunter calves were taught to drink the skim milk out of a pail, hence the term pail bunter. The calves were kept separate from the dairy cows so that they would not drink all of the milk from the dairy cows. (A good dairy cow would produce much more milk than required to feed her own calf; left on the mother, the dairy calf would "pig out" on too much milk leading to digestive upsets.)

There was always a pen of pail bunter calves beside the barn. For a time, a red-headed boy developed the habit of walking the half mile distance from town to our farm to play with me. In spite of Dad's admonishing us not to ride the pail bunter calves, we did so when Dad or other family members were not around.

My outside pants were often thread-bare or ripped. To my horror and discomfort, I developed large red patches on the insides of my legs. It was ringworm (ringworm is actually a misnomer as it is a skin infection due to a fungus). There are many different species of ringworm fungi; some species are zoonotic, that is they can spread from animals to humans via spores.

The pail bunter calves sometimes would catch "ringworm" and I caught ringworm from riding the calves. Hence my first experience with doctoring: the treatment for ringworm for both the calves and myself, was strong tincture of iodine! I still remember how badly it stung when I had to treat myself with it! (I also had to treat the calves; I think the strong tincture of iodine was a punishment for riding the calves, a more ghastly impressionable punishment than a spanking by Dad!)

As spring evolved into early summer, the dairy cows who were fed dry hay, straw, etc. over the winter months were turned out to feed upon new spring grass pasture. Usually quite lush and high in protein, the spring grass would result in the cows' manure becoming extremely loose (i.e. watery) for a while.

One Saturday, my red-headed friend, Billy Joe Green came out to our farm to play. At this time Dad still had an old barn, the dairy cows would be brought in to stand side by side in stanchion head catches to await milking. The barn had a center alleyway; behind each row of cows on either side would be a gutter to catch manure and urine. The gutters were to keep the cows' legs and udders cleaner if the cows decided to lie down.

It was a warm day so the doors to the barn were left open. Billy and I were playing cowboys and Indians; I was chasing him. He decided to run through the barn, as he ran around the corner by the barn door, he startled the closest cow who instinctively kicked, lifting poor Billy across the alleyway and into the green slosh in the gutter on that side of the barn. A cow on that side spontaneously let go a kick, sending Billy into the gutter on the other side of the barn.

I vividly recall Billy sputtering, crying, wiping at his face and running back to town. Except for a rooster tail of red hair, poor Billy Joe Green was utterly "green". That episode resulted in Billy's mother forbidding him to ever come out to our farm again!

The "ban" lasted about a month or so, when Billy made his way out to our farm again. Dad had built a "milkhouse" near our house which acted as storage for milk bottles, and it also had a cement trough. Cold water from our water well was put in the trough to keep bottles of milk cool (we had no rural power on the farm at that time, so no refrigerated coolers).

It was a hot day so Dad had a ladder up to the roof of the milkhouse and he had a pail of sticky black tar which he was applying to problem areas of the roof. A neighbor drove into the yard and requested Dad's help as some of the neighbor's cows had broken out of the fence.

Billy and I were playing tag with each other. For some reason, I ran up the ladder with Billy in hot pursuit after me. As I clamored onto the roof, I accidently kicked the bucket of tar and it went sailing, open end first onto Billy! Billy Joe Green was now "Billy Joe Black", save for the rooster tail of his red hair!

Again, Billy left for home in town, crying and screaming. That occasion absolutely marked the end to Billy coming out to the farm. I remember some of the furious "talking to" that his mother gave to my poor parents.

The schools in Bow Island were on the north side of the town, so they were the nearest part of town relative to our farm. We either walked, rode a bike or horse to school. Grade one was a rather pleasant experience probably in large part due to our very kind teacher Mrs. Meyers. I didn't know the letter B from the letter X when I first started school.

Mrs. Meyers made a fuss over each one of our birthdays. Somehow, I was smitten with the idea of my class coming out to the farm for my birthday. Mrs. Meyers and my Mom agreed to this. I was elated with the prospect of showing my classmates, the baby piglets, calves, chicks and ducklings. Sadly, it was a harsh lesson in reality for me. We were poor, our house had no running water, no power, no indoor toilet. I still can remember some of the rather horrified expressions on the faces of some of the girls in my class. My farm boy ego was deflated! The shy farm boy retreated further into the darkness of being shy.

Grade two was a rough year for me in many ways. I didn't like my grade two teacher and I think that feeling was very mutual. Instead of letting us play dodgeball, baseball or soccer, she was adamant that we should all learn tap dancing. For the boys in the class, this went over like rotting manure!

One day, I had a wrestling match with Harvey, one of my classmates; we were not fighting, we were just "horsing around". Our teacher came into the classroom, yelled at us to stop and go kneel at the front of the classroom. "You can kneel there until the hair grows on your knees" she snarled at us! Harvey and I glanced at each other and giggled. It wasn't the best thing to do as we knelt there for a very long time then. She finally relented and let us go to our desks and sit down. That was a good thing as I never did grow hair on my knees (I would still be there today)!

That year there was a couple in town who had a baby who could not tolerate cow's milk but could thrive on goat's milk. The father purchased a milking nanny goat and asked my Dad if the goat could be kept on our farm which was only a short jaunt from town where the family lived.

April 21, 1952, goes down infamously as a most terrible day in my life. Each day at that point of school, each class member had to take a textbook home, read a chapter and then give a verbal report on that chapter on the next day to the rest of the class. As it was my day to take the book home, our grade two teacher lashed out at me "Mr. Schatz, when you return this book tomorrow, I don't want to see a single black mark on any page! Do you understand Mr. Schatz?"

I ran home with the book in great excitement for that spring we had a pinto mare that Dad said was about to have a foal any day now. I tossed the book on the steps of the house and ran to the corral to see if Trixie had foaled (she hadn't yet).

Among farmers there is a truism: if your fence won't hold water, it won't hold a goat! I walked back to the house to be greeted by the horror of the nanny goat on the steps, smacking her lips. I grabbed the orange covers of the book, over 200 pages gone, neatly nibbled out by the stupid goat!

My Mom paid for the book with cream cheque money that our family really could not afford to spend for that purpose. I was in the bad books with my family for some time, later I could think to myself with some satisfaction that my teacher did not see a single black mark on any page of the book!

Some people believe in karma or something of the sort. Years later, I had obtained my driver's license and my oldest brother Everett had let me borrow his green Chev pickup truck for a while. As I was driving down main street, I spotted this cute girl wearing shorts walking down the sidewalk. The plan was to drive slowly by her, then whip around the block back to main street to hopefully ogle her beauty some more. While I was passing her for the umpteenth time, I admit that I wasn't paying too much attention to the passenger side.

At precisely the right moment, my former grade two teacher swung the door of her big Buick car to get out. I caught the edge of that door with the side of the truck bumper and snapped her car door back against the front fender of her car. As I glanced back, I still remember the horrified expression on her face, one leg and one arm suspended in mid-air. I vividly remember the white dress with purple flowers that she was wearing that day.

Her husband was a giant of a man, about 6 foot five tall. When he arrived at the scene, as a scrawny teenager, I thought I was going to die! To my intense relief he said to me, "you know she should have been watching but you could have been more careful"! I couldn't have agreed more, yes, there is a kind God.

Half a mile east of our farm was an abandoned farm site with a dense row or caragana trees along the road. Three old granaries were the only remaining buildings on this site. Its proximity to town and its seclusion made it a favorite site for teenagers to park n' spark (or whatever).

My brother Benny and I would go over to that site every Sunday, there was usually a number of empty beer bottles that we could gather up and Luke the Chinese proprietor of the Paris Café in Bow Island would reward us with candy or pop.

On one of these visits, I caught a glare coming out from between the skids of the large granary. When I investigated by reaching under the granary, I found a stash of 6 beer bottles, FULL BEER BOTTLES! As Benny and I contemplated our great find, we discussed the fact that Luke only took empty beer bottles. We decided to solve our dilemma; we drank the beer! I was about 8 and Benny was 12 years old. Our first experience getting drunk and very sick from alcohol.

Mom and Dad were not very happy with our performance with the beer. Dad said something to the effect: "the guys probably pissed in empty beer bottles and then put the caps back on and then hid them". For many years I think that discouraged us from drinking liquor. Dad could be very subtle at times.

My childhood and teenager years outside of school centered around farm chores: feeding the poultry and farm animals, cleaning manure out of pens, weeding the garden and driving Dad's Minneapolis model U tractor. I was not involved in any organized sports. At age 12 I joined the 4-H Beef Club, my project was an Angus steer calf.

Achievement (show and sale day) day was held in July in conjunction with the Medicine Hat Exhibition and Stampede. 4-H clubs from towns around Medicine Hat also participated with our Bow Island club. Our calves were kept tied up in a long green World War II former army building. We slept overnight in the straw with our calves as the exhibition lasted 3 days.

After we finished caring for our calves in the morning, we would meander through the midway grounds of the exhibition. Most of the carnival workers would sleep in late, so we walked through the idle midway rides. We discovered a bonanza: coins, pens, combs, cigarette lighters that had fallen out of the pockets of ride participants were at the bottom of the seats of the rides or on the ground below.

The midway had a large male African lion on display in a cage. One morning, 3 of us stopped in front of his cage, he was sleeping. People were starting to come into the exhibition grounds and a small crowd gathered around us by the lion cage. I suddenly had a sort of premonition and I said to my buddies "let's go". We had just worked out way out of the crowd when I turned and looked back. The lion had just stood up and I think his action was deliberate as he swung his rear end from side to side spraying the crowd as he urinated!

4-H afforded the introduction to public speaking which ultimately helped me in my veterinary career. Veterinarians need excellent communication skills with people in order to assist making a diagnosis with a sick animal.

THE FORMATIVE YEARS FOR A VETERINARIAN

The St. Mary's Irrigation District opened up in the Bow Island area in 1955 and over the succeeding years, farmers were now able to grow sugar beets, beans, potatoes, sunflowers and later corn. One year, a gentleman put out contracts for farmers to grow onions on their irrigated land. He promised to build a warehouse by fall to store, clean and bag the onions for retail sale.

That fall there was a "mountain" of onions on the site of the proposed onion plant but no building. Two of my friends, Robert and Alan, as well as myself, were contemplating the fact that frost had frozen the top layers of onions but ever changeable southern Alberta weather resulted in a warm melting spell and the once frozen onions were now balls of mush that could be thrown!

It was Halloween. Robert's father owned the John Deere/Dodge dealership on the west corner of main street. We were too old for "trick or treating" but well into the troublesome teenager years.

Robert, Alan and I filled several gunny sacks with the mushy onions. There was a trap door roof access inside of the dealership and with the aid of a tall step ladder, we took our bags of onions onto the roof. The dealership building had about a 4 foot false front to the roof which faced main street. We exhausted our supply of mushy onions by throwing them at passing cars and trucks and the poor little gremlins and goblins parading down main street.

At some point Robert's father must have come in to check his business, noticed the ladder and open roof trap door. He closed it, we were trapped on the roof and the October 31 night was starting to get very cold. The back of the building was quite tall, too high for us to jump down plus we caught a glimpse of light in the back dealership yard....some very ticked off victim(s) of our onion barrage were waiting for us to come off the roof! We went to the front of the building by main street and stated to hop over to the roof of each succeeding building on main street. A Chinese family owned a grocery store further down, we knew that they lived at the back alley end of their store. At the back of the preceding store there was a tree, it was a bit far out but Robert and I reached far out to catch a branch and then climbed down to the ground. The living area of Chuen's store sloped down to a lower height. In spite of Robert and I telling Alan to use the tree, he clamored onto the roof of Chuen's and jumped off it there.

Robert and I were further down the alley when we heard a door fly open accompanied by someone yelling in Chinese. As we dived into some bushes to try to hide, we heard the twang of a 22 caliber rifle. A branch of the bush snapped off as the bullet zoomed above our heads! We were then subjected to a barrage of gravel; Robert and I got up and ran as hard as we could. Mr. Chuen was yelling something to us in Chinese, we didn't understand a word but by his tone it was nothing complimentary to us.

Alan, the cause of all this, had hidden behind a rain barrel as soon as Mr. Chuen burst out of his door. Later Alan was calmly able to walk to his home.

Alan went on in later years to a long successful career as a Member of the Legislature of Alberta. Robert and I went on in later years to develop bad knees from our dive into the bushes!

When I wasn't working on the home farm, I spent part of the summers working for farm neighbors: John Egan, Bob Ferris, Jack Van Rousell and Joe Nixdoruf. Bob had a male Weimaraner dog Max and a female Weimaraner dog Sarah. He proposed a partnership in which I would keep Sarah and we would split the income on the sale of puppies.

At one time, the Weimaraner was a relatively new breed in Canada. Originating in Germany, this grey short haired breed was known as an excellent pointer for hunting pheasants and grouse. As a breed, they had a good disposition and friendly nature with people. My oldest brother Everett, worked for a cement and gravel business; he was able to procure used gravel screens which

THE FORMATIVE YEARS FOR A VETERINARIAN

I used to make kennels for my dog project. To my dismay (and my family), one drawback of the Weimaraner breed was the propensity to mournfully howl in the middle of the night!

Sarah developed a red mass in the medial corner of her right eye. There was no veterinarian in Bow Island at that time but a veterinarian from Medicine Hat, Dr. Stu Little, would come to Bow Island about once a week. When I took Sarah to Dr. Little, he offered to take her back to Medicine Hat, remove the "cherry eye growth" and bring her back next week. His kindness and care cemented the idea of becoming a veterinarian in my mind!

This point of my life was pivotal for I hated school in grade 9. The teacher, whether he really intended to or not, came across as rather mean and condescending. He would belittle the girl who struggled with algebra; he would even razz a student on family financial status. I don't recall exactly how many hours I spent writing out on foolscap "gentlemen do not throw chalk". He did not appreciate being hit with chalk that some of us would be throwing at classmates inside of our open window classroom. Not our fault that he walked into the classroom in the line of fire of a barrage of chalk!

I was considering quitting school at that time. My 4-H club leaders, Norvel Coffman and Dean McKnight, urged me not to quit school. "You'll never be a veterinarian if you quit school" they admonished! Norvel's wife, Iris, was my junior high English teacher and she also encouraged me a lot. Those people were great mentors for me.

High school was a big improvement. I really enjoyed chemistry 10 taught by Roy Hadlington and biology taught by Greg Johnson. Perhaps I was more mature but my grades improved somewhat. Dave Pickard was the high school principal at the time, he taught courses in math and physics. I still remember some of his great sayings: "time will pass, will you?" (great cure for daydreaming in class). Another was his explanation on averages: "if you put one foot in boiling water, and the other foot in ice old water, on the average, would you be comfortable"?

Near Bow Island, a seasonal creek (the Cherry Creek coulee) went through Dad's land just on the northwest corner of our farmyard; it also went by the eastern edge of town. One spring, the snow melt off was extremely great and the Cherry Creek rose and flowed with a great torrent of water.

My brother Benny and some of his buddies found a couple of large house-moving timbers near town. Someone had the idea to nail old board slabs to them to form a gigantic raft which was in the form of a "V". I happened to be in the tag along role of a nuisance little brother, so along with Benny and his friends, we launched the raft into the creek water. We thought we were Gods as the raft went down the Cherry Creek heading towards the South Saskatchewan River!

After about two miles, disaster struck us: a bridge on a county gravel road. The "V" shaped raft wedged under the bridge. We were "trapped" as chunks of ice and various debris started to pile up between and under the large timbers of our raft. The cold icy spring water started to rise up as our raft formed a "dam", backing up the creek water. Evening was coming and our only choice was to jump in the icy water to shore and set off for a long cold walk back home.

The County of Forty Mile probably would have dearly known who was responsible for the raft as the backed-up water eventually took out the bridge! Some things were best kept a secret at that time when we were kids.

I forget the exact year but when I was in high school, a veterinarian, Dr. Phil Bryant started a veterinary practice in Bow Island. The amiable Dr. Bryant was a great source of encouragement to me as he guided me towards the career of veterinary medicine.

Dr. Bryant's practice area covered a very broad area of southern Alberta, all the way down to the American border. He drove

THE FORMATIVE YEARS FOR A VETERINARIAN

countless miles going to farm calls! Small animal work was performed out of a couple rooms of his residence.

To his consternation, he had a spaniel dog that in spite of his best efforts, the dog developed grotesque obesity. His residence was about one block from the back alley of main street. He finally discovered that when he was away on farm calls, the dog would make trips down the back alley; the owners of the butcher shop would set out fat and various meat trimmings for the dog. No wonder Dr. Bryant's dog became overweight and a source of embarrassment as he tried to talk to small animal clients about weight issues in their pets!

During my younger years, Dad was using a threshing machine; he would set it up in the front of the big barn so that the straw could be blown into the loft of the barn. My sister, Evelyn, had a white cat with four white kittens which were her beloved pets. One day when Dad started up the tractor and engaged the belt pulley to the threshing machine there were very loud thumping sounds coming from the back of the threshing machine. Dad stopped the tractor and went to check the threshing machine; too late, the cat and kittens had crawled into the machine and the blades of the straw blower had beaten them to sacks of bones. We all felt very sorry for Evelyn, for me it was a lesson on the reality of keeping animals.

About a year later, Evelyn had a black cat who developed a rather large round growth on his nose. She named him "Bubbles" for that reason. There was no veterinarian in Bow Island and regardless spending money on a cat was not considered in those times. However, my late brother-in-law, Joe Sikora, had an idea: he proposed the use of a castrating device, the Burdizzo emasculator for lambs to remove the "bubble growth" from Bubbles' nose. The Burdizzo has two blunt jaws, when placed over the neck of the scrotum and pressed shut, it would crush the spermatic artery and vein to each testicle but it would not cut the skin of the scrotum. (In time, without a blood supply, the testicles would die and shrink up to nothing.) I held Bubbles and Joe applied the Burdizzo to the neck of the bubble growth; after the crush, Joe cut the bubble off without any bleeding of note. Bubbles recovered, Evelyn was very happy and this was another "seed" for me to become a veterinarian.

I graduated from Senator Gershaw school in Bow Island in 1963. My next step towards a career in veterinary medicine would be college!

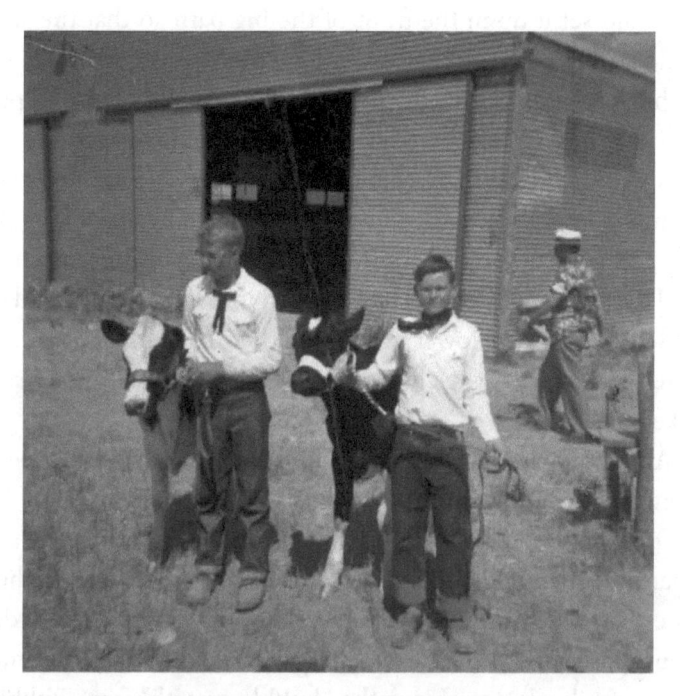

On right, Richard Martin, I'm on left with my 4H Dairy heifer

THE FORMATIVE YEARS FOR A VETERINARIAN

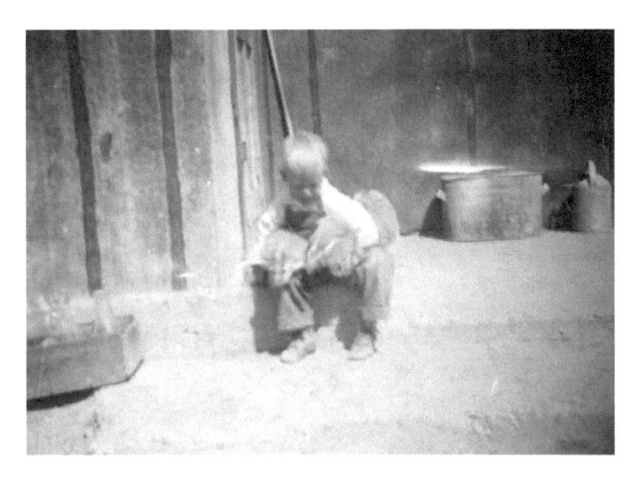

Holding the badger kits, "Bernice" and "Evelyn"

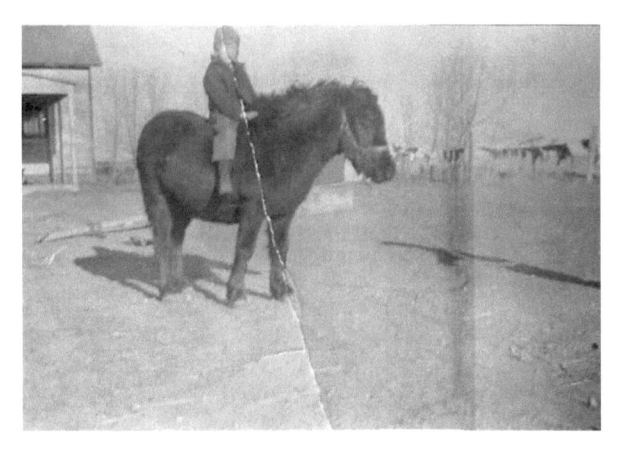

5 years old on Shetland pony "Sally". When she tired of being ridden, she bolted for a slough and laid down and rolled!

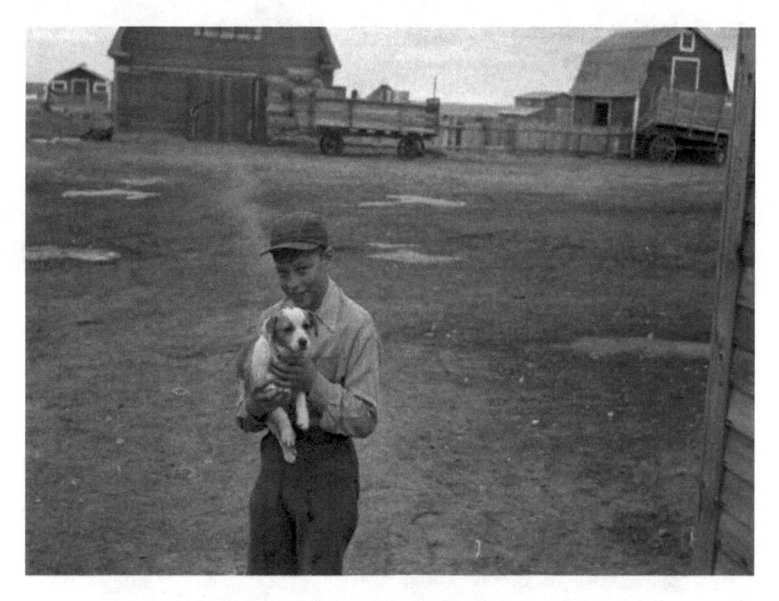

9 years old, in front of barns holding a puppy

Chapter Two

MY COLLEGE YEARS

After graduation from grade 12 in 1963, I spent most of the summer of that year working for some farm neighbors. Irrigation in the Bow Island area meant that farmers could irrigate alfalfa and often get up to 3 cuttings of alfalfa hay per summer season. At that time square bales were the norm (no large round balers yet and no New Holland automatic load bale wagons). The square bales had to be picked up by hand, hauled and stacked for winter storage and use. The pay was 3 cents per bale stacked; one hot day in the hot July sun, I hauled 1100 bales, a $33.00 pay day! Standard rate for other farm work was $5.00 per day at that time.

September of 1963, I enrolled at the Lethbridge Junior College, about one hour west of Bow Island. The college at that time, offered first year university transfer; there were 6 of us enrolled in pre-veterinary medicine. Our courses included zoology, organic chemistry, physics, English literature and even botany.

To illustrate the ravages of inflation to today, a very kindly lady, Nellie McElroy, provided room, meals and laundry for $55.00

per month! (Perhaps that was somewhat relative to a $5.00 per day summer wage.) Tuition cost as I recall was about $400.00 per session in those years.

The message was loud and clear, to be admitted to veterinary college, one had to have high grades as there was competition for limited enrollment at veterinary college. I think I applied myself with more direction than at high school and my academic performance improved.

The final exam schedule near the end of April in 1964 had the botany course as my last exam of the term. Most of the Lethbridge college students (in first year science, teaching, etc.) had their last exam on the preceding day and there was a party scheduled for the night of that day. Rather exhausted from many late nights studying for previous exams, a pre-medicine student, Jim Marfleet and I tried to focus upon studying botany. At one point Jim said "let's go to the party, we'll only stay for a little while"!

So we went to the party but the little while turned out to be a rather long while! Drinking age was 21 years, we were nineteen (should not have been drinking, a confession to my children). Our botany professor was at the party and we were aware that he was dating one of the girls at the party. In my somewhat inebriated state, jerk that I was, I started to hit upon this girl! Not a smart move but then I was never accused of high intelligence. Jim grabbed me and we somehow found our way home and crashed for a bit of sleep.

I woke up early and with the aid of a large pot of coffee, I tried to contemplate the large binder of botany notes. My plan evolved to read every 7th page (I regarded 7 as my lucky number). This I did and at the exam, there was the choice of writing short essays on 4 out of 8 botany topics! Four of those choices were topics I had just studied in detail! When I received my final grades, I calculated that I must have obtained 94% on the final botany exam!

Perhaps my whole cram study program for exams was wrong? I also wonder if I missed my calling as a botanist!

Summer break of 1964 I worked for neighboring farmer John Egan, cultivating summer fallow, putting up hay, driving grain truck, etc. September saw me off to the University of Alberta in Edmonton for my second year of pre-veterinary medicine. Students in pre-vet. medicine were in the Faculty of Agriculture with the thinking that if they were not accepted into veterinary college, they could continue on to achieve a Bachelor of Agriculture degree.

The second- year pre-vet. medicine courses included inorganic chemistry, physics, genetics, economics, public speaking and of all things: a math course, calculus with analytical geometry. I never ever applied any of that math assisting a calving cow! In retrospect, the pre-vet. medicine courses were to give us background for veterinary courses but they also tested our "mettle".

The Lister Hall residence complex was my home on campus, I shared a room with Jacob Smart, a fellow pre-vet. Medicine student. During the term, students on our floor decided to end the night with coffee, juice and lunch. Someone purchased an old toaster to make toast. The residence fire alarms started to ring at night and the city of Edmonton fire department would come rushing to the residence. Since the elevators were shut down during the fire alarm, the firemen would have to clamor up and down all 10 floors of the residence. I still vividly remember one heavy fireman in full fire fighting garb, gasp and mutter between gasps "bleep-bleep university students"! Originally the fire department thought someone was deliberately setting off the fire alarms, but it was later determined to be due to extra well-done toast!

Fall of 1964 marked the time when the maple leaf flag was scheduled to replace the Red Ensign flag of Canada. The Edmonton Jubilee auditorium was located across the street from the Lister Hall residence and there was a multitude of flag poles bearing flags. The popular escapade was to steal a Red Ensign flag as a memento.

Late one rather cold November night, two agriculture students (big Gary Smith and little Gary Smith as we called them because of their physical stature), were out attempting to steal a Red Ensign flag. Little Gary Smith had shinnied up a flagpole to take down a flag when a security guard appeared at the site. Big Gary Smith engaged the guard in what seemed an eternity of small talk while little Gary Smith shivered in the cold, trying to hide behind the flag at the top of the flagpole!

For the summer break in 1965, I worked for a small experimental farm at Oliver, just outside of Edmonton. It was a job that paid better than farm labor, important because money was always a bit of an issue during my college years.

The early sixties were an era when there was a dedicated campaign to establish a veterinary college in western Canada (Guelph, Ontario and St. Hyacinthe, Quebec were the only 2 veterinary colleges in Canada at that time). Rural areas of western Canada had a severe shortage of large animal veterinarians to serve the livestock industry.

A joint agreement among the provinces of B. C., Alberta, Saskatchewan and Manitoba was reached to fund the establishment of the Western College of Veterinary Medicine (WCVM) at the University of Saskatchewan, Saskatoon, Saskatchewan.

I applied for admission to the new veterinary college in Saskatoon and I also applied for admission to the Faculty of Medicine at the University of Alberta, Edmonton. Near the end of July 1965, I received letters of acceptance from both, a "fork in the road" for my life. As a shy, awkward farm boy, I decided that I would be more adept working with animals than being a medical doctor, dressed in suit and tie and dealing with people. I would in later years, have the revelation that good communication skills were essential to successful veterinary practice.

September of 1965 marked the beginning of 4 years of veterinary study at the U of S, Saskatoon. There were 33 of us in first year veterinary medicine, 32 "redneck" males and one "token" female, Roberta Patterson. Many of those classmates were older than me and had achieved a university degree prior to admission to veterinary college. We were a "half class" as the veterinary college building was yet to be constructed and there was only a small number of veterinary college faculty hired for the start-up college. A small building, the I.H.U. (Initial Housing Unit) had been hastily constructed. It served as a classroom and laboratory for such courses as anatomy, physiology, pharmacology, etc. We would take some first-year courses with the Faculty of Agriculture students in Kirk Hall and the agriculture building at the U of S (livestock nutrition, animal science, poultry science and range management). Another arrangement was that we would take courses in biochemistry, embryology and neuroanatomy with students in first year human medicine at the U of S.

Perhaps one of the most vivid memories of our first-year veterinary medicine, occurred on the first day, when Dr. Fraser said to us, "look at the person to your left, then look at the person to your right, when you graduate they won't be there with you!" Not sure if that remark scared me more than it made me mad. His prediction did not evolve to that degree as 27 of us out of 33 did graduate as veterinarians 4 years later.

The lone girl in our class switched to honors English even though she successfully passed the first year of veterinary medicine. It probably was very difficult being the only female in the class. This lead to our distinction as being the only all male class to graduate from the Western College of Veterinary Medicine! Today across the Colleges of Veterinary Medicine in North

America, 80-90% of the classes are female; the profession has evolved greatly.

One of our first-year veterinary medicine laboratory sessions was hematology (study of blood and its components). One lab session was on hematocrits (packed red blood cell volumes); small amounts of blood in small glass capillary tubes were spun down in a centrifuge to determine the hematocrit values.

After placement of the tubes in grooved slots in the centrifuge head, a cover was to be placed over them and screwed down before the centrifuge was turned on. One of my classmates forgot the cover; there were loud shattering sounds of tinkling as the glass capillary tubes were flung around and breaking in the centrifuge. Another of my classmates exclaimed, "what a stupid thing to do", as he flipped on the switch of his centrifuge. Again, the sound of breaking glass capillary tubes, he had made the same mistake himself! Sweet karma.

The neuroanatomy course dealt with the brain and nervous systems. There was a lecture component and a lab component to the course which was taught by professors in the Faculty of Medicine. Due to our initial class schedule, we students in veterinary medicine were not able to take part in the labs which enabled dissection of the brains of human cadavers.

Almost all of us veterinary students failed the first neuroanatomy mid-term. Dean of the Veterinary College, Dr. Larry Smith, arranged an adjustment in our class/lab schedule so that we could partake in the neuroanatomy dissection labs. It was easier to visualize parts of the brain using the cadaver specimens than just looking at one plane diagram in a textbook.

The final exam for neuroanatomy had an oral one-on-one component. Literally shaking with fear, I started the oral exam. The professor asked a question pertaining to a hemi-section area of damage to the spinal cord and what motor and sensory nerve functions would be lost. As I blurted out my limited knowledge, in my anxious state, I said "and sexual function would be lost on the left side of the body".

He laughed so hard, he literally fell off of the lab stool he was sitting on. I'm not sure if it was out of pity or out of his having a real good laugh but I did manage to pass the neuroanatomy course!

As we also shared enrollment in the embryology course with the first-year human medical students. We went for those lectures in a classroom in the medical sciences building on the U of S campus. The medical students each had their own desks (the old style with a drawer for notebooks under the seat). There were 3 female students in the human medicine class and the male students in that class also had the old "redneck male" affliction. Some of the male students in the class had removed the testicles from a cadaver in their anatomy lab and they put them in the drawer of the desk of one of the female students. This prank was verbally shared with all of the male students including those of us in veterinary medicine.

Upon entering the classroom, the female human medicine student sat down at her desk and opened the desk drawer for her embryology notes. All male eyes were upon her to watch her reaction to the testicles on top of her notebook. Without a blink of her eye, she calmly picked up the testicles, stood up and exclaimed "alright which one of you guys lost these"?

Another one of our classes we shared with the first-year human medicine students was biochemistry. The lecture portion of this course was in an amphitheater type classroom, we were sitting at the back top of this classroom. One of the biochemistry professors walked in, never spoke and just started to write on the blackboard. His writing was small and impossible to read from the back of the classroom. One of my classmates, Andy Strang, yelled out "Sir, Sir"! The professor turned around from the blackboard and Andy said "Sir, would you please write LOUDER"? Several moments silence and then the professor got the message.

Anatomy was one of our first-year veterinary courses; we had preserved specimens of cats, dogs, a horse and a cow to dissect. Dr. Eberle, our anatomy professor, was fond of telling the single members of the class that we spent too much time studying anatomy reading Playboy magazine and not enough reading Sisson and Grossman, our veterinary anatomy textbook.

Physiology (study of functioning of the body) was another major first year course, consisting of lab sessions as well as lectures. At that point in time, dogs and rats were used as terminal subjects for the labs. Our class was divided into groups of 5 or 6 students for the lab sessions. One group featured two classmates with perhaps a lackadaisical attitude (i.e. they did not graduate with the rest of us in 1969!)

One lab session involved a dog under general anesthesia. Various drugs were given during the course of the lab to demonstrate the effects of those drugs. At one point, one group's dog stopped breathing before the lab session was completed. I can still recall Dr. Dunlop, red in the face, sweating and frantically trying to administer chest massage to revive the dog. Behind Dr. Dunlop, one classmate in that group was grinning as he administered more phenobarbital in the femoral vein of the dog! If the dog died, the lab session was over… The student wanted to go to the bar! Poor Dr. Dunlop had his back towards the hind end of the dog and was unaware of the students' caper!

As a side note, I dare say that there was a time when there was a rather callous attitude in the education of medical doctors, veterinarians, lab technicians, veterinary technicians etc. as many animals were used for training labs. Today, there are many simulation aids made of rubber, plastic, etc. To reduce the use of live animals for students' education. From an animal welfare standpoint, the general attitude of what is acceptable for use of animals in education has shifted immensely. On the other hand, there is a concern that veterinary personnel will graduate with next to nothing for practical "hands on" experience with live animals.

Back to the pharmacology course, Dr. Dunlop gave us a lab assignment to conduct a "small drug research project" of our own design. This was an era in time when gas anesthetic drugs (such as halothane and methoxyflorane) were just being introduced to veterinary medicine. The old standard of introducing a state of "sedation/anesthesia" in cattle and sheep was a drug, chloral hydrate, which could be given intravenously. At one time chloral hydrate was used as an oral tablet in human medicine as a treatment for insomnia and some types of seizures.

My group decided that one would put an ewe (female sheep) "down" with chloral hydrate and then give her a newly licensed respiratory stimulant drug Dopram (Doxapram hydrochloride) to see if it would shorten the recovery time from the chloral hydrate "anesthesia". An overdose of chloral hydrate could induce respiratory failure.

We put a catheter in the jugular vein of the ewe and started to administer the chloral hydrate solution intravenously. After a while as expected, the ewe laid down on the I.H.U. floor. The plan was to get her to a "heavy" plane of anesthesia and then give her the Dopram. However, the ewe started to struggle to get back up; one of us knelt over the ewe to keep her down while more chloral hydrate was given. Alas, the ewe just kept trying to stand up.

Very perplexed, we called Dr. Dunlop over. He told me that sometimes a drug idiosyncrasy (abnormal or unexpected physical reaction to a drug) could occur and that we could write up our lab report as an example of drug idiosyncrasy.

After he left, we let the ewe stand up and then we realized that the ewe had laid down catheter side down over the area of the floor drain. The I.V. tubing had disconnected and all of the chloral hydrate solution was going D.T.D. (Down the drain).

Our dilemma was whether or not we should confess to basic stupidity or to write the lab report as a drug idiosyncrasy!

We did not have any further classes with the contemporary human medical students after our first year. Similar to us, the human medical students had a pharmacology course in their second year.

One of the pharmacology lab sessions involved injecting a series of drugs at varying doses into members of the class to demonstrate the affects of the drugs. For example, a dose of atropine lending to dilation of the pupils of the eye and "dry mouth".

There was a member of the human medical class who was disliked and ostracized by the rest of the class. In our era, he was called a "square", among today's young people I think the term is a "nerd".

The pharmacology professor stepped out of the lab for a while. At this point, some of the lab group strayed from the prescribed lab protocol and injected the "square" with a non-prescribed drug: succinylcholine.

Succinylcholine causes body muscles to go into a state of relaxation. Fully conscious under this drug, the poor "square" turned blue as he struggled to breathe while mentally freaking out. The lab group mates pretended not to notice him for some period of time until they finally relented and gave him a reversing drug (neostigmine) for the succinylcholine.

Needless to say, the human medicine faculty responded with severe punishment for the perpetrators of that very dangerous prank! (i.e. I think their year of graduation was extended by one year.)

On a side note, there was a period of time (about 60 years ago) when some veterinarians used succinylcholine for horse castrations. An injection of succinylcholine would cause the stud horse to fall down, immobilized for a while; the horse could then be castrated. There is no analgesic (i.e. pain killing) effect to succinylcholine, so the horse had pain during the operation! Thankfully today we have effective anesthetic/analgesic drugs for horse castration and post-op alleviation of pain.

We often referred to ourselves as the "guinea pig class" as our professors were rushed to develop courses for the first class of the Western College of Veterinary Medicine. Our final exam in physiology started at 8:00 a.m. and as the day progressed, just when we thought we were done writing, either Dr. Roe or Dr. Dunlop would come in with yet another exam question. Many of us were still there after 5:00 p.m. in the afternoon still writing but some had left "early" for the consolation of the Executive House bar!

Construction of the main building for WCVM commenced but then a major glitch was discovered; the site featured an underground aquifer. The construction company pulled off the job for additional piles would need to be placed to support the building properly. Poor Dean Smith had to seek additional funding from the university to get the construction company back on the job. This resulted in a delay of the main building of WCVM; our class would have access to this building near the end of our third year and even in our fourth-year construction of some areas was still occurring.

I'm not sure what compelled me, but I undertook to put out a monthly class newsletter, The Probe, for the supposed edification and entertainment of my classmates. (I had some experience with our school newsletter, The Venture, when I was in high school in Bow Island.)

The summer of 1966, I spent in Edmonton as I had found a summer job with the Faculty of Agriculture at the University of Alberta. Dr. Grieve arranged a tour up to the Peace Country of northern Alberta, little did I ever imagine that I would ever end up living there later in my career.

Some of the second-year veterinary courses were parasitology, pharmacology and pathology. There was a research building (the

Fulton Lab) on the U of S campus, and it was connected by an underground tunnel to a Veterinary Hygiene building. These buildings were next to the site of the WCVM building.

The Fulton Lab was a center for research into a number of diseases which could infect humans as well as animals. Western Equine Encephalomyelitis (sleeping sickness) was one of these diseases. There was a small post-mortem (autopsy) room in the Fulton lab as well as lab rooms. Our pathology professors improvised and made accommodations to deal with limited space. Our class recalls benches set up in the tunnel so that pathology specimens could be put out for practical pathology exams. We squeezed by each other and just made do. Pathology toughened out stomachs as not all specimens were in a "fresh state"!

The centennial year summer of 1967 was spent employed by the Health of Animals Branch, Canadian Department of Agriculture. First half of that summer was spent in Vancouver, B.C. and involved work in meat inspection at various packing plants (cattle, pig, sheep and poultry). Second half of that summer employment was out in the Fraser Valley near Langley. Health of Animal veterinarians were at that time still quite involved with T.B. (tuberculosis) testing of cattle and also brucellosis[18] testing of cattle. The intent of the employment was to entice veterinary students to work for the government upon graduation; I decided being a government veterinarian was not for me.

Third year of veterinary college involved courses such as radiology, livestock and small animal diseases, clinical pathology and introductory surgery. We had been joined by succeeding year classes (class of 1970 and class of 1971), so some of our lecture classes were still in Kirk Hall and other U of S buildings. Happily, some of the new WCVM building was available for classes for the winter of 1968 session.

The veterinary college purchased the veterinary practice (in Saskatoon) of Drs. Gavin Hamilton and Ted Clark so that veterinary students could learn from actual clinical cases that were attended to by staff veterinarians.

In the summer of 1968, four of us were selected to work for the veterinary college for our summer employment. We would do rotations through the small animal clinic, large animal clinic and ambulatory calls (farm). The University of Saskatchewan operated and maintained a laboratory animal building to provide research animals for research projects related to human medicine, nutrition, pharmacological studies, etc. In collaboration with the veterinary college, there was a project to have a new strain of mice delivered by sterile Cesarean section to be "germ free". The black mouse colony harbored a bacterial infection, pseudomonas, the existing white mouse strain within the U of S laboratory colony was free of that bacterial infection. Some of the genetic make-up of the black mouse strain made it more suitable for certain research projects over the genetic make-up of the white mouse strain. The intent of the project was to introduce the black mouse strain into the laboratory facility without contamination of the existing white mouse colony.

For 6 weeks of the summer, one of the 4 of us would work on the "mouse project"; the 4 of us decided to draw straws…..I lost. Many "germ-free" baby mice were "delivered" by me and a lab technician. Once delivered the idea was that they would be suckled by the pseudomonas free white strain mouse mothers. To our great disappointment, the fostering aspect of the project was a total failure as none of the fostered black strain germ-free baby mice survived! I decided that a career as a laboratory animal veterinarian was not for me. I also regretted that I "lost out" of the experiences the other 3 of my classmates had with early summer calving cases, foaling cases, etc.

Fourth year of veterinary medicine marked all of our classes and labs in the new veterinary college building although there were still some uncompleted areas. In addition to the classes of

'70 and '71 we were joined by the class of '72. The completion of construction of WCVM would enable the admission of a full class (60) veterinary students in September.

In groups of 3 or 4 students, we had rotations through radiology, surgery, clinic and farm calls, as well as more lecture courses. A new large animal surgery professor, Dr. Larry Kramer, was hired and one night most of our class were in a Saskatoon bar with him. He was a giant of a man, about 6 foot four and about 300 pounds. Maybe it was just the beer or maybe just my poor judgement, but I passed a package of the bar peanuts to him and said, "would you like some peanuts"? "No", he snapped. I responded with "oh excuse me, I thought I was feeding the elephant"! That certainly did not put me in his good graces!

When we returned for our final session in January of 1969, the large animal medicine professor, Dr. Otto Radostits came into our classroom and started to tell us about the number of rural large animal veterinarians who were leaving their practices for work as small animal veterinarians or for employment as government veterinarians. For many years, veterinarians had been able to earn a substantial amount of their yearly income vaccinating heifer calves for a disease brucellosis[18], that caused abortions in cattle. The federal government paid $1.00 per calf vaccinated and tagged with records to be filed. Vaccination for brucellosis was not 100% effective but along with a test and slaughter program for adult cattle, Canada was able to move from an infection rate of 30% of the national cattle herd to an infection rate of about 0.05% of the Canadian herd. Brucellosis could cause major economic loss due to cattle aborting and it could also cause a serious disease of humans (undulant fever).

The federal government decided that the level of brucellosis was so low that the mandatory vaccination of heifer calves would be discontinued in 1969 but farmers could continue (at their own cost) to have their calves vaccinated for brucellosis.

MY COLLEGE YEARS

None the less this new policy would alter large animal practice in western Canada.

In retrospect, I wish that I was more mature or more resilient, but I took Dr. Radostits' prediction of gloom and doom for beef cattle practice too seriously as I became discouraged and "slacked off" in my studies in that final session.

Being a homely, shy and awkward farm boy, I only had a few dates with girls to that point of my life. There were several female students in the class of 1972 at WCVM and somehow as we crossed paths by the WCVM library, I caught the eye of one of these female students (or vice versa). She invited me to attend a Joni Mitchell concert in Saskatoon with her and thus began my first serious relationship with a girl. As I will relate later, it was the start of an unsuccessful relationship but one that would occasion a major shift in my life and career.

I and a classmate of mine, Rex Benoit, had developed friendships with three members of the class of 1971: Warren Weber, Dave Lightfoot and Gord Davis. After a night of studying at the university library (or an empty classroom), we would cap the night off with a snack at one of the fast-food drive-in restaurants on 8th street in Saskatoon. As the Saskatoon winter waned in early April of 1969, some guy would have his buddies drive him around these fast-food joints and this guy would "moon" the patrons! The 8th street "mooner" became rather infamous. We were at the A & W parking lot when the mooner made his appearance. A very quick-witted Warren Weber, jerked our car door open, and threw his mug of hot chocolate on the exposed posterior of the "mooner"! Needless to say, there were no more reports of sightings of the "8th street mooner" after that!

As my last session at WCVM was approaching, I had decided that the dairy cattle industry was more stable than the beef cattle industry at that time. Through one of the faculty professors, I made contact with Dr. Jim Vandevelde of Abbotsford, B.C. He wanted to hire an associate veterinarian and I agreed to join him after I graduated. I was somewhat familiar with the Fraser Valley of B.C. as I had worked there during my summer job of 1967. There were numerous dairy farms in the Fraser Valley to supply milk for the city of Vancouver.

This seemed like a good decision for my career in veterinary medicine but at this time I was also as "twitterpated" as a 15 year old teenager with my girlfriend who would be continuing her studies at WCVM. Probably not too realistic but we would agree to a "long distance" relationship while I went to work in B.C.

The end of April 1969 marked the end of my 6 year quest to become a veterinarian, one of 27 successful survivors for the class of 1969 at WCVM!

Based on my newly acquired degree, the Bank of Nova Scotia gave me a loan of $3600 with which I was able to purchase a brand new Mercury Montego car.

MY COLLEGE YEARS

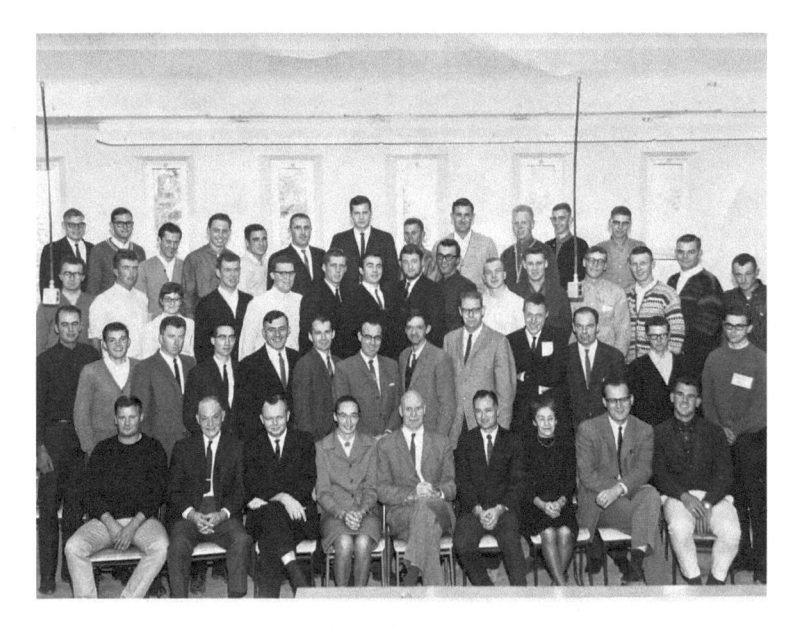

Western College of Veterinary Medicine
Faculty and First Class September 1965

(left to right)

Back row: Lawrence Ford, Ernest Olfert, Jim Hanson, Graham Hickling, Bob Gainer, Ross Clark, Don Jamieson, Bob Hope, Terry Church, Dick Krauss, Andy Strang, Grant Maxie

3rd row: Rex Benoit, Al Sutton, Roberta Paterson, Pete Rempel, Albert Anderson, Gordon MacKenzie, Doug Baker, Jon Sector, Jacob Smart, Ed Neufeld, Paul Edwards, Art Schatz, Wayne Burwash, Doug Graham, Gary Quamme

2nd row: Edward Wiebe, Dick Weetman, Dr. Red Fraser, Dr. Bob Clugston, Dr. Bob Dunlop, Dr. Saunders, Dr. Chris Bigland, Dr. Allen, Dr. Herb Carlson, Dr. Ole Nielsen, Dr. Walter Roe, Gary Harbin, Pat Brennan.

Front row: Bob Evenson, Dr. John Milton, Dr. Eberle, College Librarian, Dean Larry Smith, Dr. Bill Cates, Dr. Jean Murray, Dr. Otto Radostits, Al Matheson

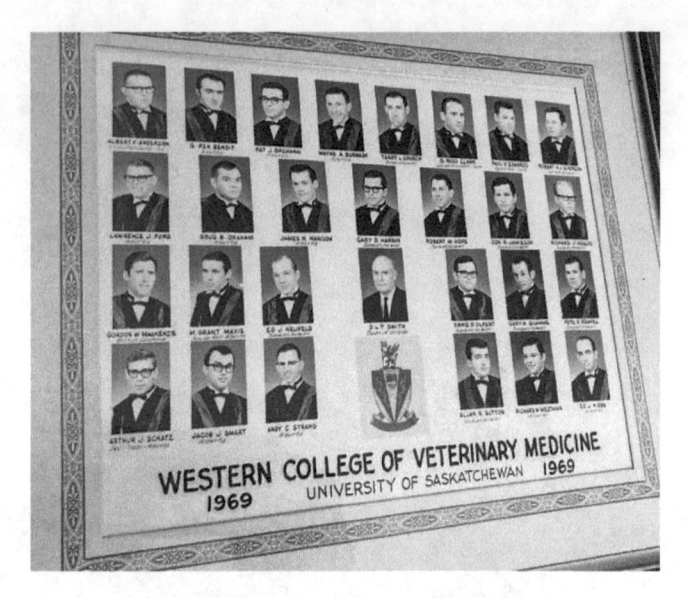

First Graduation class of WCVM 1969!

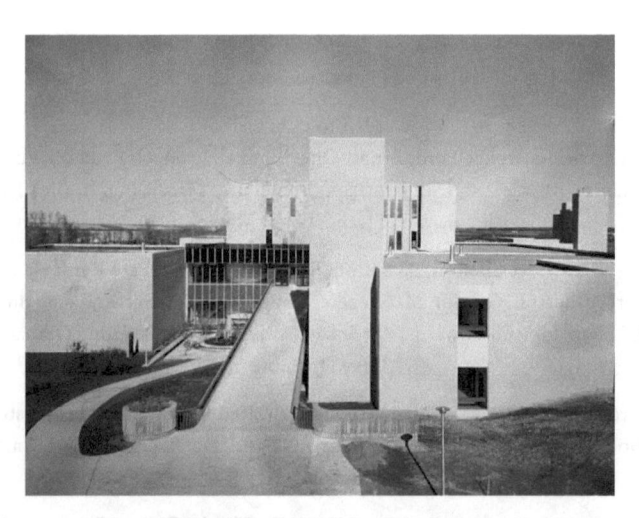

Completed College of Veterinary Medicine 1969
University of Saskatchewan. Saskatoon, Saskatchewan.

Chapter Three

VETERINARY PRACTICE: THE FIRST HALF YEAR!

I had about a month of free time after graduation before starting employment in Abbottsford, B.C. Time for a bit of relaxation time to visit Mom and Dad on the farm and also a few more dates with my girlfriend before saying goodbyes.

Dr. Vandevelde was a 1962 graduate of the Ontario Veterinary College, and he started a solo mixed practice in Abbotsford. He had a building constructed on Ware Road, that had small animal facilities on the main floor and living quarters for himself and his young family on the second floor. The large animal portion of the practice work was performed by doing farm calls. I was able to obtain room and board with the kindly Scott Hines family in Abbottsford.

The small animal position of the practice consisted mostly of vaccinations and neuters of dogs and cats. I didn't mind the small animal work but as a new graduate, I had big visions of "helping feed the world" by serving food animal production.

Dr. Vandevelde served as a mentor for me for the regular office hours of veterinary practice but it was a rather rude awakening to be on my own for evening and weekend calls. At veterinary college there was always a college professor and fellow students to confer with over cases; now as a young "green" graduate, I had to deal with the application of knowledge to the practical aspects of veterinary practice (often under the critical eyes of the animal owner)!

Many veterinary practices at that time did not have an x-ray machine or if one were available, it would be something of an antique cast off from a human hospital or chiropractic practice. Likewise, blood work and blood chemistry tests were not available as at veterinary college. As a new veterinarian to achieve a diagnosis, one had to rely on the history from the owner and a physical examination of the animal. Dr. Radostits had left us with this poignant saying "more things are missed by not looking than by not knowing"! However, I wished I had paid more attention to some classes.

I am always proud of the fact that the term "to vet" the legal document or insurance policy arose because veterinarians became known for thorough physical examinations. That being said, veterinary medicine is not immune from errors in diagnosis, treatment or surgery. Even in human medicine (although equipped with better diagnostic equipment and lab tests) thousands of human deaths occur in North America each year due to errors in diagnosis, treatment or surgery. An older veterinarian once said to me "you'll establish a cemetery in your first year of practice".

There was an opportunity to cater to horse work in Dr. Vandevelde's practice and this was presented to me. A client who worked all day at a sawmill had an 8 year-old Palomino stallion.

VETERINARY PRACTICE: THE FIRST HALF YEAR!

The client had an acreage, and the stallion was getting out and creating havoc for neighbors who had geldings or mares. Since the client had decided to have the stallion castrated, I was asked to come out in the evening when the client was home from work.

An appointment was thus made for a July evening for me to come out and castrate the stallion. As a veterinary student at college, I had the opportunity to castrate one horse before I graduated. At that time, the standard in veterinary practice was to anesthetize the horse with an injection of a "short acting" barbiturate.

I gave the stallion the injection and when he went down, I tied the upper hind leg forward, scrubbed and disinfected the scrotal skin and performed the surgical castration. A routine injection of tetanus anti-toxin and one of "long acting" penicillin was given to the "new gelding".

A major problem of the barbiturate anesthesia was a "stormy recovery": the horse would try to stand up before it had regained the "placement reflexes for its feet". One had to sit on the horse's neck, hold the head bent back and try to keep the horse down longer, otherwise the horse would stumble, fall over and potentially damage itself in the recovery from the anesthetic.

To this point, the castration had gone well and although the horse struggled a fair bit, I managed to get him standing up. I was about to leave when I decided that since the stallion was "quite maturely developed", I should look under his belly to check for untoward bleeding.

To my immense horror there was a loop of small intestine protruding from one of the castration incisions! This "herniation" of small intestine can be a rare occurrence following castration. The testicles of a male embryo foal form within the abdominal cavity and as they are suspended by long spermatic artery, vein, nerve and spermatic cord they descend (drop through a small opening (inguinal ring)) in the ventral abdominal muscles into the scrotal sac. Intestines in the scrotum is known as a scrotal hernia. It can have a hereditary basis where the inguinal ring is larger than normal, however, it may occur to heavy exertion such as a "stormy" recovery from the barbiturate anesthetic.

The "norm" for equine castrations was to leave the surgical incisions open (i.e. not sutured) to allow for post-op drainage and prevent post-op swelling. Intestine hanging out of an open incision was a major catastrophe ; the protrusion of intestine would become more and more progressive with more loops coming out. I had heard a story from an older veterinarian who also had this unfortunate experience; in his case, the horse panicked, began kicking at his belly, struck a hoof through a loop of intestine and literally tore its own guts out before dying!

In a panic, I put the horse down again with another barbiturate injection and rolled him on his back. By this time, there was a considerable amount of intestine protruding out! I was not prepared for this event; I did not have a large amount of sterile saline to wash the intestines before replacement, I had no sterile drapes, gauze packing, etc. to deal with this emergency situation!

The intestine was thus lying on the hair of the horse's belly (gross contamination) and also to my dismay, a zillion flies were also using the exposed intestine as a landing site!

With "sweat pouring down the crack of my ischial tuberosity" on that hot July evening, (as I was frantically pushing the intestines back through the inguinal ring into the abdominal cavity), a crowd of people had gathered on the other side of the corral fence. I still recall a sweet little old lady proclaiming very loudly "I've seen thousands of horses castrated and that's never happened! He sure must have done something wrong"!

I finally got the intestines replaced and fortunately had some suture material with me to suture the inguinal ring opening shut. After another long while, I was able to get the horse recovered from the anesthetic and standing up. It was not a great feeling as certainly there was a lot of contamination of the intestines and there would be a huge chance of a generalized infection of the inside of the abdominal cavity (peritonitis) occurring which could be fatal. Another concern was that in the process of replacing the intestines, I could have inadvertently caused a twist in them. This could also have fatal consequences.

At that time there were few drugs available for visceral pain relief, the only option I had was phenylbutazone as a post-op pain killer for the horse. I also gave him more penicillin (a rather massive dose) as the big concern would be infection developing.

Sick at heart and devastated, I slept a very sleepless night worrying. Next day, I went out to check on the horse 3 times; he was not eating but temperature, pulse rate were only slightly elevated. On the second day post-op, he was holding steady but still not eating. The owner phoned me early on the morning of the third day post-op and said, "he's eating this morning"!

I didn't have a chance to check on the horse until late on the third afternoon. When I went into the stable, I found him dead on the stable floor!

There was a fox farm nearby and the owner had him delivered there. When I performed the autopsy, there was scant peritonitis but the horse evidently feeling better had consumed most of a square hay bale and bucket of oats…..a condition called gastric dilation and torsion (extreme swelling and twisting of the stomach) had occurred and the stomach had ruptured causing death!

I felt like the material on the bottom of a septic tank. My profession was supposed to be about preventing suffering and saving animal's lives. My inexperience had resulted in my not being prepared with having suitable materials and drugs with me. I had also failed to "twig" (even though I saw the full manger of hay and oats) on the possibility of the horse over-eating.

So much for my being the "great horse veterinarian" for the practice, as news tends to travel fast among horse owners.

I did manage to pull myself together and castrate quite a number of horses in later years of my career. A hard lesson had been learned: when out on a country call always be well prepared. On 2 other occasions of horse castrations in future practice, I had intestinal herniation occur, but I was prepared and able to successfully save those 2 cases. Fortunately, also in later years, improved anesthetic drugs and painkillers became available for equine practice.

Needless to say, this incident left me rather depressed for some time. Suicide of veterinarians is an issue for the profession in today's world; it was also an issue over 50 years ago. That summer, I learned of the suicide of one of my college professors, a man I thought had everything going for him. There is the frustration of losing cases, the frustration of having cases for which there is no treatment or cure, the frustration of some client's ignorance and uncaring, the frustration of clients not being able to pay for veterinary care, the frustration of managing a business, frustration of dealing with difficult people and a frustrating toll on the family of a veterinarian. Counselling was not available to any degree fifty-five years ago, certainly there are now more resources to help professionals with mental health but yet suicide of veterinarians is still a sad reality.

Summer of 1969 marked man landing on the moon, I still recall watching that event on television. In my off-time, I was able to entertain myself by attending the Abbotsford Air Show and a couple of football games at Empire Stadium. At that time a younger guy (that I knew from Bow Island school years) was a member of the RCMP stationed in Abbotsford. One night he invited me to come along with several other off-duty RCMP members for a night in a bar in Bellingham, Washington (just across the border from Abbotsford).

A number of young local Abbotsford males were in the bar and some of them had grudges for the RCMP members (for

VETERINARY PRACTICE: THE FIRST HALF YEAR!

speeding tickets, etc.)......a brawl broke out between these two parties. I thought that it was amusing for the RCMP (and myself) to be escorted back to the US/Canada border by American state troopers!

Another interesting aside, one day I was treating a dairy cow with milk fever (low blood calcium) for a Canadian farmer whose property adjoined the American border (south of Abbotsford). I asked the Canadian farmer what it was like having an American "next door" farmer. "Well, he replied, the American keeps a rifle by his front door and a shotgun by his back door". I asked him why and the American said "you never know when a Commie or a black will come to your door"! The attitudes and prejudices of various societies are most definitely affected by our schools and media from one country to another!

My girlfriend and I corresponded with letters and phone calls that summer. She flew out to Vancouver in August and stayed in a spare room at the Hines' residence. We enjoyed a trip to Vancouver Island and touring Victoria. After the horse castration disaster, her visit made me feel happier.

She flew out for another visit that fall however, I should have sensed that things were not the same between us. We had our first argument over a silly movie. After that she did not write as often. The writing was on the wall, but I refused to read and comprehend it.

Through a classmate, I heard that Dr. Knudsen in Wetaskiwin, Alberta was interested in hiring a veterinarian. By this time, I had decided that I should relocate to be closer to my girlfriend who was back attending the veterinary college in Saskatoon. I contacted Dr. Knudsen, he had already hired a veterinarian but referred me to Dr. Keith Leitch of Wainwright, Alberta. Dr. Leitch accepted my application, and I gave notice of my resignation to Dr. Vandevelde. Wainwright was about a four-hour drive to Saskatoon and also about a four-hour drive south to my parents. The move back to Alberta seemed like the right thing to do to preserve the relationship with my girlfriend. It was to be a monumental change in the direction of my life. From a financial standpoint it was probably a dumb decision for if I had stayed in that area of B.C. and invested in real estate there, the return would have been astronomical.

I drove back to Alberta just before Christmas day and upon visiting my girlfriend, she gave me the "big goodbye"! Christmas was spent with my parents and sibling's families. On New Year's Day, 1970, I drove to Wainwright to start my employment with Dr. Leitch.

Chapter Four

A TRIBUTE TO DR. LEITCH

The Wainwright and surrounding areas had veterinary service since the early 1900's by a Dr. Wiley, a Dr. St. Jean and a Dr. Farley until the late 1940's.

Dr. J.M. (Max) Saville was a World War II veteran. After the war, he enrolled in the Ontario Veterinary College. Upon graduation in 1949, he set up practice in Chauvin, Alberta and then moved to Wainwright four years later.

There were few veterinary practices in Western Canada and Dr. Saville covered a large area of Alberta. He wore out many cars travelling on muddy or snow filled roads. Sometimes he would be taken to an animal by horse and wagon or horse and sleigh. Few farms or ranches had cattle handling facilities in those days so veterinary practice for Dr. Saville was very physically demanding and often dangerous.

Dr. Saville built one of the first veterinary clinics in Alberta for large animal service which was officially opened on October 5th, 1963. The concept was very successful in that area as the farmers and ranchers quickly adapted to hauling their sick animals to the clinic. This saved the veterinarian hours of time that was previously spent driving and increased the service provided for more clients.

Dr. Keith Leitch graduated from the Ontario Veterinary College in 1962. He practiced for a while in Saskatchewan. One of his stories is going to a farm call in his old Volkswagen accompanied by his Alsatian Shephard dog. After attending to a sick cow, he and the farmer returned to the fact that in the meantime, his dog had killed several of the farmer's chickens. Keith's $5.00 call charge was quickly reversed to compensate for the dead chickens! Rural Veterinary medicine has had a long history of not being very lucrative for veterinarians!

Dr. Leitch joined Dr. Saville's practice in February of 1963. The clinic building was under construction at that time. Dr. Saville and his wife, Lil, operated the veterinary practice out of their home and at times Keith recalls scouring (diarrhea) calves brought to the house for treatment. Keith also recalled answering the door of Dr. Saville's house and the client asked, "is your daddy home"?

Keith met Dianne Herauf in 1964, and they were married January 23, 1965. Their family consisted of Ed, David, Michael and Kelly as the years progressed. Keith purchased the practice from Dr. Saville in 1967, and Dr. Saville went on to serve as a Field Veterinarian with the B.C. Department of Agriculture. Drs. James Rowe, Dennis Hughes, Robert Bourne and Kim McKellar worked with Dr. Leitch in the next few years. Dr. Art Schatz joined the practice January 1, 1970, and purchased a share of the clinic in 1971.

For many years in the late 1950's and the 1960's, the mainstay for economic survival of rural veterinarians in western Canada was the compulsory vaccination program for heifer (female) calves for a disease called brucellosis. This disease caused abortions and reproductive problems in cattle and a serious disease called undulant fever in humans. The vaccination program lasted 2 to 3 months every fall, with the government paying the veterinarian $1.00 per calf vaccinated.

Keith told of one occasion when he was on a farm. It was about -30 degrees and getting dark. The farmer had about twenty extremely wild black Angus heifer calves for vaccination in a very old barn. There was no cattle chute or squeeze; one had to crowd the calves up to vaccinate and tag them. At one end of the barn was a very dilapidated barn door and the farmer stood in front of this door to keep the calves from bursting out. The calves churned about as Keith tried to perform his task and at one point the calves hit a support post in the barn and broke it off….the post had a couple of sets of old work horse harnesses on it and the post and harnesses landed on top of Keith!

The calves ran for the door, the farmer yelled at them, and they turned back and ran and jumped over Keith as he struggled to extricate himself from the tangled harness (this occurred a number of times). Keith said, "for a while, all I could remember was black hooves, black bellies and black teats"!

Dr. Keith Leitch was extremely well liked by clients of the clinic. His soft-spoken but sincere manner won their complete trust. Perhaps some of Keith's adoration by people may have been due to the fact that Dr. Saville had at times a rough and caustic manner. One client related the time when Dr. Saville went out to a calving at the farmer's place on a hot day in July. The calf was in a posterior breech presentation (coming butt first with the hindlegs doubled forward underneath the calf's body). Since the cow had been trying to calve for a while before the farmer found her, the calf had died in utero (womb) and was starting to decompose (i.e. becoming rotten and very smelly)!

Dr. Saville sat up on the top corral rail with a mickey of whiskey and snarled directions to the farmer as to how to manipulate the calf's body and legs so that the malpresentation could be corrected and then the calf delivered. As the farmer completed the task, gasping for breath and covered in sweat and gore, Dr. Saville walked over to him and gave him a bill for "consultation"!

(This story was told to me years later and the farmer was still sputtering about Dr. Saville!)

My future father and mother-in-law told the story about an evening call by Dr. Saville to treat a dairy cow with milk fever (low blood calcium level). Luke invited Dr. Saville in for a drink.... Luke was a staunch Irish catholic and Dr. Saville loved to argue religion, politics or for that matter, that black was white. Kathleen (my mother-in-law) states that the night began with a 26 ounce bottle of whiskey on the kitchen table, Max (a protestant) and Luke (a Catholic), deep in argument.

Kathleen went to bed, leaving the 2 men locked in fierce debate. In the morning when she got up, Dr. Saville was gone as were all of the contents of the whiskey bottle! (My wife claims that her Dad would only have had one shot glass of the whiskey!)

However, in spite of a few quirks of Dr. Saville, there is no doubt that he worked very hard to provide veterinary service. He practiced for some time in an era when antibiotics, other antimicrobial drugs, newer anesthetic drugs, etc. were not available. This was also in a time when there were "laymen animal doctors" in the ranching and farming communities. Veterinarians were few and far between in western Canada so as a trained veterinarian, he faced the hurtle of educating clientele about nutrition and husbandry of livestock. Dr. Saville showed an envisionary spirit of entrepreneurship when he built the veterinary clinic in Wainwright; it became a model for other veterinary clinic buildings in western Canada.

During most of Dr. Saville's years of practice, if a calf could not be delivered by manual assistance (i.e. pulling), the choices were to euthanize the mother cow then cut the calf out of her body or to deliver the calf by a fetotomy. (Sometimes erroneously called an embryotomy.) This was the procedure of cutting the calf's body into smaller parts so that delivery could be accomplished. In some cases, the difficult decision to euthanize a live calf was made before doing a fetotomy. Dr. Saville was said to have a legendary skill of using a wheel wrench (the pointed end served as a chisel) to perform a fetotomy.

When Dr. Leitch arrived in Wainwright, he amazed (and impressed) local farmers and ranchers because he performed Caesarian sections on cows, saving the lives of both the cows and their calves.

The procedure of Caesarean section was known to be possible during the fifties, however, post-operative infections rendered most of these Caesareans impractical due to death of the cows by infection. Dr. Leitch took his veterinary training at a time when penicillin became licensed for veterinary use and newer improved local anesthetic drugs became available. As a recent veterinary graduate, Dr. Leitch was able to bring the new advances to veterinary practice. Dr. Saville was readily converted to performing Caesareans after observing Dr. Leitch's successes with the procedure.

In February of 1970, a farmer brought in a very sick shorthorn heifer to Wainwright veterinary clinic. Examination revealed that she had an emphysematous calf in her uterus and was becoming very toxic. (Emphysematous refers to the condition where the dead body is decomposing i.e. rotting and various bacteria produce gas in the process.) The emphysema (gas) causes the affected carcass to swell up and also become very odoriferous!!

The first choice procedure would have been to perform a fetotomy to deliver the emphysematous calf. However, the heifer's cervix was only dilated 3 fingers open, so it was impossible to reach into the uterus to do a fetotomy. Another choice would have been to euthanize the heifer for humane reasons. A third choice was to perform a midline Caesarean. (Most commonly a Caesarean section on a cow is performed with the surgical incision done on the left flank abdominal region with the cow standing up.)

For the midline Caesarean procedure, the cow is cast (pulled down with ropes) and rolled up on her back; feet and legs tied forward and back. The ventral abdomen is clipped and scrubbed to allow for a long surgical incision to be made on the midline of the abdomen.

Since the body of the emphysematous calf is usually very greatly swollen up, the midline Caesarean creates more room for delivery. In addition, the approach allows more of the pregnant horn of the cow's uterus to be brought outside of the abdomen. When the uterus is incised to deliver the emphysematous calf it also allows for infected fluid and debris to drain outside of the peritoneal (abdominal) cavity of the cow, preventing a fatal peritonitis/infection of the abdominal organs from developing (in spite of antibiotic treatment).

Upon discussion with the farmer, Keith (Dr. Leitch) and I proceeded with the midline Caesarean. Our receptionist, Bella Ford, allowed a number of clients who just had questions to come to the large animal area of the clinic as both of us were involved with the surgery. One of these clients made the macho-man comment, "this is the operation a pregnant woman should be watching".

When Keith cut into the wall of the exposed uterus, several gallons of dirty, smelly, rotten fluid poured onto the clinic floor. I heard the sound of someone throwing up...."macho-man" was by the overhead door of the clinic, attempting to get out (which he did after several bouts of throwing up).

We did not have any assistant that day, so the body of the rotten calf was left on the clinic floor while Keith and I sutured up the incisions. At the point where we were about finished, "macho-man" had got over being sick, had made his way to the front of the clinic. He had not previously asked his questions, so as he peeped his head through the door to the large animal room, Keith spotted him. With a twinkle in his eyes, Keith exclaimed "dammit George, if you had blown into it's mouth, we could have saved it"!

A gag and macho-man disappeared again!

The coffee room of the Wainwright Veterinary Clinic was the site of revitalization for the veterinarians and staff. It faced south to the street and at night, the lights in the coffee room served as a beacon for clients, friends and sometimes an adjournment site after the local bars closed.

Calving season in 1971 seemed to drag on forever probably as a result of the "exotic cattle boom". The "exotic" breeds of cattle (such as Simmental, Charolais, Maine Anjou and Limousin) were being introduced to north America because these breeds were noted for rapid growth rates. Prices for the exotics were very high compared to the local British breeds of cattle (Aberdeen Angus, Hereford and Shorthorn). Cattlemen were using A.I. (artificial insemination) breeding of local cattle to the exotic breeds of cattle. The trait of rapid growth rate was manifested by the large size many of these crossbred calves developed during pregnancy. As a result, dystocia (difficulty giving birth) became a rather rampant problem and as veterinarians we were called upon to assist (which meant an increase in the number of Caesareans performed by veterinarians).

Dr. Leitch and I were literally kept going 24/7 all spring. In the middle of the night on a day late in May, we were both waiting in the coffee room for the next cases to arrive at the clinic. A truck pulled up and 2 of the locals, very loud and quite obviously a bit inebriated staggered into the coffee room. One of them was holding his head to one side and moaning and groaning in apparent pain.

"Dr. Leitch, you've got to help-s me, there's a fly stuck in my ear-sh", he wailed. A twinkle developed in Keith's (Dr. Leitch) eyes, he grinned and said, "alright John, hold on". Keith went to the exam room and reappeared with a 20 cc plastic syringe. Keith flashed his other hand to me to reveal a dead fly which he had fortuitously found somewhere.

"Hold your head more to that side John", said Keith. While holding the closed hand with the dead fly next to John's right ear, Keith blew a bit of air in the syringe into John's left ear.

Keith whipped his closed hand in front of John's face; opened his palm to reveal the dead fly and said "look John, I blew it out the other side"! There was a moment or two of silence, a look of some consternation, and then a broad smile appeared on John's face.

"Keith", John said, "your-sh the best doctor in town, I feel okay now"! After thanking Keith several times, John and his happy buddy staggered out into the night.

Dr. Keith Leitch was not only the best doctor in town, he was also the one with the quickest wit and greatest sense of humor!

Most of the Caesarean sections performed by veterinarians are due to fetal (calf) oversize compared to the size of the boney pelvic canal of the cow. There are a number of reasons for this problem: 1) first birth heifers that have not been sufficiently grown out before breeding (nutrition and age are factors here), 2) the introduction of the large exotic breeds of cattle which were bred to our "native", smaller British breeds of cattle, 3) a deformed pelvis of the dam (mother), 4) prolonged gestation (pregnancy) length resulting in higher birth weight calves.

However, besides "size 5 calf, size 2 mother", Caesareans are sometimes required to deliver severely deformed calves that cannot be delivered by vaginal birth. Examples of these deformities include cases of Siamese (conjoined) twins, two-headed calves, various extra legs, arthrogryposis and schistosumus reflexes to name just a few. These deformities may have various causes; genetic, nutritional, poison or chemical toxicity and "unknown".

Arthrogryposis is a condition in which the calf forms with a twisted curved spine and the legs are crooked with joints that do not flex (bend). There may be various internal defects in the calf's body organs as well. An early issue in the days of the first exotic breeds of cattle was the fact that some of them were carriers of a recessive gene for the arthrogryposis complex; when 2 carriers of this recessive gene were bred, an arthrogryposis calf could develop. Not to be rather uncharitable but when Canadian farmers first went to Europe to select exotic breed cattle to import to Canada (at high prices), the European farmers who knew the problem carrier bloodlines, unloaded these problem bloodlines onto the unsuspecting Canadian farmers. This may have increased veterinary business, but it was a costly learning process for the Canadian cattle industry! Instead of being worth $20,000, $30,000 or even more at birth, the dead full blood arthrogryptic calf was "literally a dead loss"!

In the condition, schistosumus reflexes, the calf's body is essentially formed turned "inside out". The pregnancy usually progresses to term; the calf's rib cage and abdominal wall does not join at the ventral midline of the calf's body. This results in the heart, lungs and abdominal organs being literally dangling out in the open and the 4 legs are directed backwards (opposite direction) to the abdominal organs. This type of deformed calf is usually impossible to deliver by vaginal birth because the body of the calf is locked in the state of "rigidity". As veterinarians we can assist the birth of a schistosumus reflexes calf by performing either a fetotomy or a Caesarean.

One busy spring evening, Keith and I were both busy with incoming clients and their animals. A very grim-faced farmer unloaded a Hereford cow with four calf hooves protruding out the lips of her vulva. The farmer said to Keith, "I've been working on her for hours, I can't push it back to get either the 2 front legs or the 2 hind legs to come. I can feel the head to the right side and I'm sure that it's not twins".

Keith performed a vaginal examination on the cow and with a twinkle in his eye, glanced over to me and said, "I'll have to do a Caesarean, Bill". I was busy treating a chilled out (hypothermic) calf when Keith called me over to pull the calf out of the cow's uterus. I dropped the schistosomus reflexes calf onto the clinic floor. As Bill gazed at it in amazement, Keith said to him "Bill, you pushed so hard on it, you pushed it's guts out"! Poor Bill's face turned red, and he let out a groan.

After this bit of subtle Dr. Keith Leitch humor, he proceeded to explain the schistosomus reflexes condition to Bill, pointing out the fact that it had a recessive gene cause.

The convenience of the veterinary clinic did not eliminate all farm calls; there was still the requirement for farm calls for herd work, cases such as a prolapsed uterus, a downer cow, etc. (i.e. an animal which could not walk).

As demanding as large animal practice was during the early 1970's and the exotic cattle boom, it was also very demanding for the veterinarian's wife and family. Lil Saville, Dianne Leitch and my wife Eileen, not only had to contend with a crying baby during the night, they also had their sleep interrupted by farmers calling in the middle of the night for a veterinarian who was already out on a call. The heroic wives performed an answering service in days when regular telephone service was not always reliable (no cell phones, mobile phones, etc. in those days).

For veterinarians in solo large animal practice, sometimes the wife bundled the kids up and drove the car so the exhausted veterinarian husband could catch up on a bit of sleep. Sometimes we wondered if we would survive but somehow, we did survive!

A TRIBUTE TO DR. LEITCH

A great advance in our practice was the advent of an answering service provided by a local lady, Donna Harris. Donna took night calls for the veterinary clinic, the local medical doctors, natural gas company, power company, fire department, some oilfield companies and the local RCMP. She once told me "Art, you and Keith get more night calls than all of the others combined"!

A neighboring veterinarian, the late Dr. Glen Weir, of Lloydminster, Alberta was a great prankster. On more than one occasion, (not in the calving season though), Keith or I would get a call in the middle of the night.....Dr. Weir was extremely good at mimicking the accent of a Ukrainian farmer, Swedish farmer, French farmer, etc. in regard to an emergency. I admit Dr. Weir fooled me a time or two.

For some of the breeders of purebred cattle, they did not like it if a veterinarian decided to perform a Caesarean on their cow or heifer. Having an animal or more with Caesarean scars made their pitch of "easy calving bloodlines" a hard sell to prospective buyers of purebred bulls.

Dr. Weir had one such client who did not want him to do a Caesarean. This was the time when Elastoplast tape became available for veterinary use. "Look", said Dr. Weir, "there's this new tape which will hold the skin so tight together, in three-weeks time when you pull the tape off, there will be no scar whatsoever"! "There will be no stitch scars", persuaded Dr. Weir. The client reluctantly agreed and went to a local bar for a while.

Dr. Weir was able to deliver the calf without having to do a Caesarean. To illustrate the prankster side of Dr. Weir, the heifer's side was shaved as if she had surgery and Dr. Weir applied a strip of Elastoplast tape where the "non Caesarean" was performed. Three weeks later, the client came back very excited...."Doc, there was absolutely no scar at all"! After some minutes of amusement Dr. Weir explained the ruse to the client! (He had billed the client for a Caesarean which helped him sell his prank.)

I was a very quiet shy farm boy and I choose to become a veterinarian rather than a medical doctor because I would be dealing with animals rather than people. Oh boy, did I ever have a steep learning curve….fortunately successful, gregarious veterinarians such as Dr. Leitch (and also Dr. Weir) demonstrated their amazing people skills to me. Regardless of one's skills in surgery or diagnostics, it is the personality of the veterinarian which builds the trust and loyalty of clients!

Veterinary college is a fine place to acquire knowledge but it did not teach me the real art of veterinary practice…..people skills. Over the years our practice employed a number of veterinarians, summer practicum students and animal health technologists. With his quiet manner and unlimited patience, Dr. Leitch was an outstanding mentor and teacher. If someone did screw up, Keith would not correct or admonish someone in front of a client or other staff; he would quietly take that person aside to a private place and have a quiet "corrective" talk.

In the fall of 1972 to the spring of 1973, Dr. Leitch was asked to work as a visiting practitioner at the Western College of Veterinary Medicine in Saskatoon, Saskatchewan. His patience and practical manner won the hearts of the veterinary students and at the end of his tenure, he was given the award, "Professor of the Year" by votes of the students.

A further honor for Dr. Leitch occurred in 1990. The Alberta Veterinary Medical Association gave him the award "Veterinarian of the Year". This was in recognition of his years of veterinary practice service, involvement with the veterinary association and his many years of service in community organizations (rodeo association, minor hockey, 4-H, baseball and feeder's associations).

The late Dr. Leitch was an outstanding credit to his profession, his family and community.

There were some disadvantages to a large animal veterinary clinic: sometimes the animal the farmer brought in was not really a true representation of the rest of the affected animals on the farm. Another disadvantage or problem was that just as the waiting room of a human medical clinic, there always the potential of disease transmission in spite of one's best efforts to wash down and disinfect from one farmer's animal to another farmer's animal.

A third problem with a large animal clinic was the occasional escape! For some years, as veterinarians, some of the cases presented were pigs with umbilical (naval area) hernias and scrotal hernias (intestines in the scrotal sac along with the testicles). These hernias could be corrected by surgery.

Dr. Bill Crawford worked in our practice for over a year. One hot July day, he and our assistant had a number of pig hernia cases to operate on and one boisterous pig slipped out of Chuck Hutchinson's grasp and bolted out the open clinic door. Poor Chuck, in high rubber boots (i.e. no running shoes) ran after the pig which ran onto highway 14 with Chuck in hot pursuit! The pig decided to run east at full speed down the center line of the highway, past the Husky Gasliner Café. (The local coffee crowd observed this all and had their best laugh of the year!)

In the meantime, Dr. Crawford had jumped in one of the clinic cars and joined Chuck down the highway in pursuit of the pig. Further down the highway was a seed cleaning plant and next to it the local auto wreckers (with several acres of old vehicle bodies). Fortunately, there were a few farmers talking outside of the seed cleaning plant, Dr. Crawford yelled out to them "$10.00 to the man that catches that pig". The pig (and also Chuck) was by now somewhat exhausted, and one farmer managed to catch it.

At that time the clinic charge was $10.00 for the hernia repair on the pig. Like I mentioned previously, large animal veterinary practice was not lucrative in those years.

In the early 1970's, a number of farmers and ranchers had stock (horse) trailers to haul their animals to the veterinary clinic. However, many were still hauling their animals in half-ton trucks or grain trucks with stock racks. Some of these stock racks were made of wood and to put it mildly, very flimsy!

One day a farmer brought in a yearling (year old) Simmental bull for a "semen test" (evaluation of semen and breeding soundness). The bull was in a pick-up truck with wood stock racks; the ride to town and being away from other cattle put the bull into an excited "frenzy" wild state. When the farmer backed up to the unloading chute ramp at our clinic, he had backed up off-center, leaving a space between the end of the loading chute and the side of his truck box. The farmer took the back gate out of the stock racks at which point, the now crazy wild bull charged out of that space (instead of going down the unloading chute ramp)!

The bull galloped out of our clinic yard, half charging at a couple of cars, then across the highway and into some bush beside the local golf course. Past experience had taught Keith and I that as long as a crazy mad cow or bull was headed out of town and away from people, that the best course of action was not to give chase but to let the animal find its way to cattle on a neighboring farm.

Sure enough, 2 days later, my brothers-in-law who ran a dairy farm 2 miles north of Wainwright reported that the Simmental bull was in with their Holstein dairy cows. Fortunately, he had become calmer, and his owner borrowed a horse trailer and picked the bull up at the in-law's dairy farm.

I guess the farmer was somewhat disconcerted because he never attempted to risk another escape at the veterinary clinic for the bull's semen test.

About 9 months later, my brother-in-law showed me a white faced black calf with large Simmental like ears which his very top producing registered Holstein cow had just given birth to....the bull was a proven breeder!

Another escapee from our veterinary clinic was a registered purebred horned Hereford cow. In cattle practice, a relatively common occurrence was a type of cancer (squamous cell carcinoma), commonly known as cancer eye because it often occurs on the eyeball and/or surrounding tissues. This type of cancer is malignant and will metastasize (spread) to other areas of the body. (Humans and other species may sometimes develop this type of cancer.)

Predisposing factors to development of this type of cancer are unpigmented skin (i.e. pink) around the eye, ultraviolet rays in sunlight, age of the animal and irritation (i.e. dust, face flies, etc.). The condition may occur in all breeds of cattle but those breeds with a white face (for example Hereford) are somewhat more susceptible.

Treatments are varied and may include electrocautery, lazer, radioactive gold implants and surgery. Cases with a small lesion may be trimmed out by surgery but if the lesion is deemed rather large and extensive, an enucleation of the eye (complete removal of the eye) may be performed by a veterinarian.

Dr. Leitch had performed an eye enucleation on the Hereford cow and when he and the owner turned her out to the loading chute to the farmer's truck, the truck rolled forward a bit from the loading chute.

The cow seized this opportunity and went out the open space. She must have wanted to see a movie or visit a restaurant in downtown Wainwright as she headed south down main street!

Meanwhile Dr. Leitch and the farmer ran back into the clinic and grabbed a lariat rope and a halter. They ran after the cow and Keith was able to place the lariat rope around her horns. The cow was not really wild but she was very determined to keep going south down main street. Keith and the farmer were trying to lead her back to the clinic as cars stopped and by-standers on the street cheered them (or the cow) on! Some helpful men did join them and they all managed to push and pull the cow back to the veterinary clinic.

For many years, the majority of the Wainwright Veterinary Clinic work was large animal but we also had small animal cases. Dr. Saville had allowed for in the construction of the clinic, a small animal examination room, a small animal surgery room and a kennel room on the main floor. There was a partial basement under the clinic, some of which, included a kitchen room, bedroom and sitting room area.

Dr. Leitch lived in this basement suite for a while after the clinic opened. However convenient to work, the basement suite turned out to be a rather bad idea. After the local bars shut down for the night, Keith was often the object of someone ringing the clinic doorbell in the middle of the night. Most of the men who came to the clinic in the middle of the night were quite happy and also quite persistent. The thought that they needed a bottle of medicine or just to talk about a cow that acted strange 5 years ago were among the reasons for their "emergency night calls"!

Needless to say, there were nights when poor Dr. Leitch really needed to catch up on some sleep and did not need the rather frivolous night clinic consultations by clients. I do feel that many of them did take advantage of Keith's endless good nature!

After marrying Dianne, Keith bought a house in Wainwright. Going into my second year of practice in Wainwright, we decided to convert the downstairs living suite into a small animal surgery, small animal treatment room and a kennel room for dogs and cats. (The upstairs small animal surgery room was converted to a radiology room (x-ray machine, etc.) and the upstairs kennel room was converted to a post-mortem (autopsy) room.)

The kitchen room had a counter with sink and cupboards; at the end of the counter by the wall was a kitchen stove. The stove

A TRIBUTE TO DR. LEITCH

was moved out and sold off, leaving that area of the counter as an open space. The refrigerator was also moved out leaving room for a small animal surgery table and a gas anesthetic machine.

One day, Dr. Leitch and assistant June Fountain were about to perform an ovariohysterectomy (spay) operation on a long-haired black female cat belonging to one of the local medical doctors, Dr. Ian Forrester. As Dr. Leitch and June were about to administer the anesthetic, the cat had a "hissy fit", bit and scratched June, escaped and bolted from the treatment room to the surgery room (former kitchen).

At the end of the counter (where the kitchen stove once was) the cat ran in that corner; there was the open 4-inch high space under the counter which the cat found as a hiding place. Opening the bottom counter doors and thumping on the counter floor did not flush the cat out. Dr. Leitch had the idea to take an electric drill, drill a hole in the counter floor and then cut out a hole with a saw so that one could reach in and either grab the cat or flush it out the open end of the counter.

"Whir, whir" went the drill and a loud meow-meow followed; the cat went streaking out the other end. Dr. Leitch and June were then able to corner and capture the cat and finally do the spay operation. However, Dr. Leitch had the awkward (and rather embarrassing) task of explaining to Dr. Forrester why his pet cat had a spot of missing black hair and a skin abrasion on the middle of the cat's back!! Dr. Forrester took it all in good humor with a laugh. "You know", he told Keith, "we sometimes have human patients who try to escape from the hospital"!

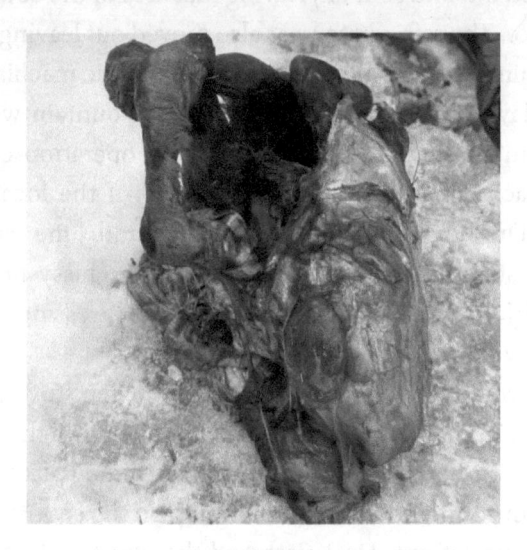

Schistosomus reflexus deformity in a calf

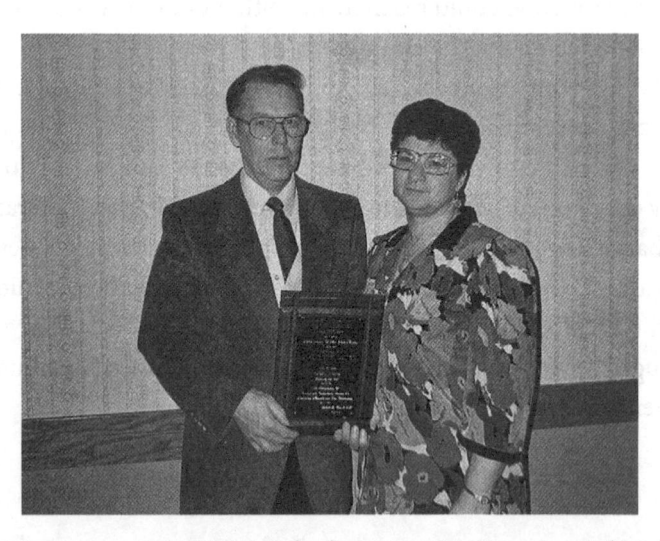

My late partner Dr. Keith Leitch (left) with his wife Dianne Leitch (right).
Alberta Veterinary Medical Association Veterinarian of the Year Award 1990.

Chapter Five

RABIES

Fall/winter of 1970-71 was noted for a high incidence of rabies[13] in wildlife in Alberta, and needless to say, positive cases of rabies were being recorded by veterinary practices.

Beware of the "mad dog" (which ran around drooling saliva and biting people or other animals at will) has been recorded for hundreds of years of human history. Rabies is a very serious disease if contacted by a human; with all the advances in human medicine there are (to my knowledge) only 2 known cases of humans surviving rabies (with exhaustive modern medicine). The disease is endemic in many countries and hundreds of human deaths due to rabies still occur annually in those countries. It is highly fatal in most mammalian species, but it is believed that skunks and bats can be inapparent carriers.

This disease is caused by a virus and transmission of the virus usually occurs through the bite of an infected animal to another animal or a person (the virus is secreted into the saliva of the affected animal). In more recent years, it has been shown that the rabies virus can be transmitted by aerosol (in the air) and through the conjunctiva of the eyes.

The virus affects the brain and nervous system with death eventually being due to paralysis. In veterinary medicine, we often refer to a furious form (mad dog) of rabies and a dumb form. Dogs and cats most often get the furious form while cattle most often get the dumb form.

One day in November of 1970, a farmer brought a yearling roan Shorthorn heifer to our clinic. She was having trouble using her hindlegs, not very steady and drooling saliva. I could not see any sores in her mouth nor determine any problem with her spine. My most likely diagnosis was rabies and since our clinic had an isolation ward, I hospitalized her for further observation. I warned the farmer that she would likely go on to die of rabies and told him to watch the rest of his herd carefully.

I elected to give her "shotgun treatments": vitamin A injection for vitamin A deficiency, vitamin B1 (thiamine) for polioencephalmacia (a brain affliction) and tetracycline (antibiotic) for a bacterial brain infection called listeriosis. To my immense surprise, over the next 5 days, she regained control of her hindlegs, the salivation stopped, and she started to eat well.

As I was helping the farmer walk her up the loading ramp to his pickup truck to take her home, he kept poking me with his elbow and repeating "rabies, eh" several times.

About 1 week later, I was out doing some farm calls in the area where he lived. He had left a message to stop in at his farm; he had a downer cow (cow that couldn't stand up).

When I examined his red Shorthorn cow, my probable diagnosis was the dumb form of rabies. As I was telling the farmer this, he was just rolling his eyes (I'm sure he was thinking "dumb green veterinarian"). I warned him and his family not to put bare hands (i.e. wear plastic or rubber gloves) if they handled her in any way. As I was leaving, I told him that if she died to let me know and

RABIES

I would come out and do a post-mortem (autopsy) so that the brain could be submitted to the federal laboratory in Lethbridge for rabies testing. Positive diagnosis of rabies was based upon histopathological (microscopic examination) examination of brain tissue and a mouse inoculation test during that era of time.

Two days later, I just happened to be out on a call in his area. I hadn't heard from him, but I decided to drop in and check on his down cow. He wasn't home and when I went out to the corral, I found that the cow had probably just died. The weather at this time was running -20C degrees to -30C degrees daily. Since the carcass wasn't frozen solid yet, I proceeded to do a post-mortem. It was late in the December afternoon, and I had to use the headlights of the car for light.

Shivering with cold and with numb hands, as I opened her up, I could not find any obvious gross lesions in her internal organs, etc. I cut her head off to put in a plastic bag to take back to our clinic where the brain could be removed. Half frozen I stumbled on a frozen lump of cow manure and as I fell, the exposed cut end of the cow's head sloshed a bit of blood in my face! Not a good thing if the cow should turn out to be positive for rabies.

Later back at the clinic, I removed the cow's brain and had it sent to the federal lab for rabies testing. Several days later, I got a phone call: the test was positive for Rabies!!

When a positive case of rabies is diagnosed, human public health departments are notified to assess the possible degree of human exposure. The farmer revealed that he had ignored my advice and had put a stick in the cow's mouth to get her "to get her cud back". Sick ruminant animals such as cows regurgitate feed that they have gobbled up in a hurry and when they are resting, they chew the regurgitated feed (the cud) into finer material for easier digestion. When sick for many reasons, a cow will stop chewing her cud; we say that rumination has stopped (i.e. lost her cud).

The farmer had put the stick in the cow's mouth without wearing rubber gloves (against my advice) so he would have had exposure to the cow's saliva. Public health officials ordered him to have the preventative rabies treatment (Pasteur treatment) which consisted of a series of injections into the abdominal muscles. This treatment was somewhat painful and there was the risk that certain individuals could have a type of anaphylactic (allergic) reaction to the treatment. The farmer was one of those individuals…..his body swelled up and he became very ill for some time. Fortunately, he survived this reaction, and he did not develop rabies!

I also had possible exposure (the blood splashed in my face) but while students at veterinary college we had received one of the first human vaccines for rabies. After vaccination we were tested for protective antibody levels for rabies protection. I had tested well, for a high level of protective antibodies so the public health officials decided that I should just receive a booster vaccination for my "exposure". (I did not require the dreaded Pasteur treatment.)

The booster vaccination was given by Dr. Vic Sawchuk at our local human medical clinic. Just as a nurse was drawing up the dose of vaccine, he said to her "use a smaller gauge needle, he's like one of us"!

I confess that in the following weeks, I did worry if my vaccinations were protective and if I would develop rabies. (The incubation period to development of rabies from the point of exposure has been known to be as long as 6 months.)

In retrospect, I often wonder about the yearling Shorthorn heifer, did she actually have rabies and recover? We were taught that once signs of rabies appeared, the afflicted individual would progress on to die. There was no cure or recovery. Is our level of knowledge correct in this regard? I regret that an antibody test on the "recovered" Shorthorn heifer was not done in the following months and when I thought about it, she had been sold and could not be traced. Experts in the rabies field will no doubt scoff at the possibility that she was a recovered case of rabies, but I wonder. Was her case merely coincidental relative to the positive case?

As an aside, in light of the rabies scare of 1970-71, the provincial government instituted a program of trapping and euthanizing skunks in an effort to reduce one of the perceived main reservoirs harboring the rabies virus. When we moved to the Peace country of Alberta in 1987, we discovered that there were no skunks around, the depopulation program was very successful in some areas! Only in the last few months have I heard of skunk sightings in our Peace country region.

A further note: when I was in practice at Abbottsford, B.C., we were asked by clients to descent young skunk kits as the vogue was for people to have pet skunks. At that time, we used a ball of cotton soaked with ether as the method of anesthesia for removal of the scent glands. Needless to say, one was very careful not to puncture or nick the scent glands during the surgical removal of them! One elderly couple had a pet skunk, it turned out to be extremely jealous if the husband sat close to the wife; it would then bite him! Needless to say, that pet was given away!

Alberta has a regulation that skunks cannot be kept as pets because of the danger of rabies transmission. In 1969, B.C. did not have such a regulation, so that was why skunk de-scenting was one of my early veterinary practice experiences.

Chapter Six

BOOM AND BUST

When I arrived in Wainwright on New Year's day 1970, I confess that I was very down-hearted after the Christmas "farewell" from my girlfriend. Dr. Leitch and his wife Dianne met me with open arms, a delicious meal, and 2 (or 3 or 4) drinks of rum. I felt better later on that day!

Dr. Leitch found room and board for me provided by a very kindly lady, Mrs. Katie Gartner. It was an eye-opener for me to work out of a large veterinary clinic that had large animal stalls, large animal head gate and examination area as well as a large reception room and also small examine room, surgery and kennel room.

It was about 1 year ago since Dr. Radostits had made his dire speech about large animal practice in western Canada. 1970 marked the beginning of the "exotic boom" for the beef cattle industry in Canada. The Federal Minister of Agriculture, Harry Hays had worked through a protocol of testing, isolation of imported cattle from Europe. During the 1950's and 1960's, a line of thinking had developed in the beef cattle show rings of Canada and the U.S. A.; the "ideal beef animal" was a short stubby block. This lead to a progressive down sizing of the existing British beef breeds in Canada (Hereford, Angus and Shorthorn). It also lead to dwarfism and poor rates of gain of weight (leading to poor financial returns).

The European continental breeds such as Charolais, Simmental, Limousin, Gelbvieh and Maine Anjou were noted for rapid rate of gain. A very serious disease (foot and mouth disease) was endemic in Europe. This disease which is caused by a virus could inflict serious economic loss in cattle, swine and sheep due to erosions and ulcers in the mouth and digestive tract; because of pain, the afflicted animals would stop eating, loose weight and could die. Canada was free of foot and mouth disease and had control processes to prevent the causative virus from being introduced into Canada.

By opening up the importation of the exotic breeds, the Canadian beef industry had hopes of greater return due to improved weight gains. Once cleared for Canada, bull semen could be collected and used for artificial insemination of existing Canadian cattle to the exotic cattle breeds. This spurred prices for the beef cattle industry, also at this time, stock market returns on the Toronto stock market were poor. Investors turned to the exotic cattle and prices of beef cattle started to soar in 1970. One result was that with more valuable cattle, farmers were more likely to seek veterinary services.

At this time the new technology of embryo transfer was also being developed. It allowed for the possibility of collecting many embryos from a valuable purebred cow and the possibility of her producing many more calves in her lifetime than by natural breeding/gestation cycles. This further added to the boom in the cattle industry!

All of this meant that many calving problems developed when our existing cattle were bred to the larger fast growing exotic breeds. I recall getting back to our clinic after doing a farm call; there was a line-up of trucks and horse trailers at the clinic going down the street and part way down main street. At times Keith and I thought that we would never get through all the cases.

The exotic cattle boom lead to a dramatic increase in the number of Caesarean sections performed by veterinarians in the early 1970's. Our practice peaked at 500 in 1973 and in addition we dealt with about 300 assisted deliveries of calves where no bovine Caesarian was required!

Along with all the spring obstetrical cases, we dealt with myriads of sick calves; scours, (diarrhea), pneumonia, broken legs, etc. This was also the time of year when we performed many breeding soundness (evaluation of bull semen as well as physical breeding potential) examinations. Among all of this we had small animal cases, swine cases, horse cases and a bit of poultry work.

By the time June rolled around, Keith and I were literally "walking zombies" (totally exhausted). We lost weight during the spring calving seasons!

In 1971, Keith and I decided to have a large addition made to our veterinary clinic; it allowed space for 2 more headgate areas, a post-mortem room, a new larger isolation ward and more large animal stalls. During the early 1970's, we were able to hire a number of new veterinary graduates to assist us. In early 1974, we had 3 associate veterinarians working for us, and we thought that "veterinary life" was good.

The high cattle prices at that time lead, of course, to a high price of beef at the meat counter for consumers. Then disaster struck…..President Nixon of the United States put a ceiling cap on the price of beef! (No American president ever put a cap on the price of oil though.) For cattle farmers, the bottom fell out of the live cattle market.

This drastically affected our predominantly beef cattle practice, as our cattle work plummeted. Most farmers were not willing to seek veterinary services for a hundred-dollar cow during this time. Keith and I could no longer afford to keep our hired veterinarians. Indeed we were now faced with keeping up the mortgage payments for our clinic building, for several months we literally drew no personal wages to keep things going. For a spell, our wives' employment bought groceries for our families.

Our veterinary practice as with the beef cattle industry had gone from boom to bust. A harsh reality for large animal veterinary practices in western Canada throughout the years was the ups and downs of the beef cycle. It has been one of the reasons for the large animal veterinarians shortage. The impetus for starting the Western College of Veterinary Medicine was the shortage of rural cattle veterinarians; fast forward from the mid 1960's to today and the shortage of rural cattle veterinarians is still a problem in Canada.

Chapter Seven

NARCOLEPSY AND FATIGUE

June 1970, Warren Webber was employed as a senior veterinary student in our practice and one evening he invited me over for coffee and a visit. While sitting and talking with Warren and his wife Mavis, I inexplicitly and rudely fell asleep. Warren jolted me awake as he had thrown a wet dish cloth in my face. Embarrassed, I tried to write this incident off as due to being exhausted at the end of calving season.

Over the years, I experienced sudden bouts of this falling asleep behavior at inappropriate times and circumstances. I would always rationalize this behavior as oh well, due to the night call, the strenuous calving case, etc. My situation became of more concern and embarrassment when I attended our veterinary conventions; I would fall asleep during the continuing education seminars. I just could not help myself; I often was the source of amusement to my fellow veterinarians as they would watch me fall asleep and wake with a head jerk!

Things seemed to slowly progress to the point where I started to doze off while driving. Summer of 1987, I was returning from a late-night country call. Suddenly I glanced out the window and muttered to myself, "what are all the cattails doing on the road"? I had fallen asleep, driven off the road into a slough with cattails.

Safety of myself and my family had now become a concern and I worried about how long I could keep going in practice. In July of 1987, I noticed an ad in the Edmonton Journal: there was an opening for a veterinarian as an instructor in the Animal Health Technology Program, Fairview College, Fairview, Alberta.

Somewhat intrigued by this ad, I had the thought that with regular day work hours and no night calls, I might cope better. I thought that a change of pace would be good for me.

That July (1987) we made a trip to a friend's cabin at Germundson's Landing, B.C. and on the way, we took a northern route that went through Fairview, Alberta. It was an opportunity to tour Fairview College and mull over whether or not to apply for the instructor position there. Our trip back home to Wainwright was memorable as we just missed going through Edmonton when the terrible tornado struck parts of that city on July 31, 1987.

One of my main concerns in making the decision to apply for the instructor position at Fairview College was locating a veterinarian to work in my place in our Wainwright veterinary practice as I did not want to "abandon" my partner, Dr. Leitch, and our associate veterinarian, Dr. Tannis Tupper.

After many phone calls and inquiries, I was able to contact a veterinarian, Dr. Heine Paulsen (a former native of Wainwright) who was quite willing to relocate from Saskatchewan back to Alberta. That issue being addressed, I formally applied for the instructor position at Fairview. I was called for an interview in early September and offered the position. I confess I

NARCOLEPSY AND FATIGUE

vacillated back and forth quite a bit before I accepted the offer of the position.

My arrangement was that I would take a one year leave of absence from practice at that time. I started work at Fairview College in late September, classes had already started about the first week of September. Eileen and the kids were left with the task of packing our belongings, some for the move to Fairview and the rest were packed for storage in the basement of our Wainwright home.

I was able to rent an acreage northeast of Fairview and on October 23, 1987 we moved to Fairview. In the topper of my Ford pick-up, our 4 kids were happy with 8 rabbits, two cats, our Golden Retrievers (Ole and Rusty) and their 10 puppies. Behind the truck, I pulled the horse trailer with a loaded deep freeze, cabinet and our 2 horses. Eileen drove the station wagon and our dear friends Barry and Yvonne Godwin accompanied us with his grain truck filled with some of our belongings.

The one year "leave of absence" from veterinary practice evolved into many years as in 1988, I was offered (and accepted) tenure at Fairview College.

Over the years working for the College, I was able to cope fairly well with no night calls or long hours as when I was in veterinary practice. I still had the bouts of uncontrollable "sleeping spells" but I was managing. For many years I did the typical guy thing and did not see a doctor. When I started to consult medical doctors, they could not determine the cause of my narcolepsy and fatigue. One doctor even suggested that it was all in my head. (I knew he had the wrong diagnosis for there's nothing in my head!)

In 2006, there was a new doctor from South Africa in Fairview. In my visit with him, he was actually spending some time looking at my medical records on computer. "You know", he said, "you are somewhat anemic, and you've been so for some time". He referred me for a bone marrow tap in Grande Prairie.

At this time, I would have an eight o'clock class and would have to go to my office and put my head down for a ten-minute rest between classes. I also started to develop nose bleeds, which I never had a problem with in previous years. My fatigue was becoming worse as was the frequency of my sleeping spells.

I finally had the bone marrow tap; the result was a bit startling: aplastic anemia! Aplastic anemia means that the bone marrow has stopped making red blood cells, white cells and platelets. It is regarded as a serious diagnosis, potentially fatal and the treatment would be a bone marrow transplant. As an aside in the bone marrow report pathology was one line; there is one cell which has a "hairy cell" appearance.

For many years, there was an antibiotic, chloramphenicol, which was widely used in both human and veterinary medicine. Once deemed safe, in later years it was discovered that about 1 in 50 people would react to this antibiotic and develop aplastic anemia. I certainly had a few spills when filling a syringe with the antibiotic and leakage onto my skin. Some "safe things" are learned the hard way not to be safe in both human and veterinary medicine. A coffee room trick was to sneak a drop of chloramphenicol into a co-worker's coffee; it produced a very bitter taste in one's mouth and profuse salivation.

My family doctor and I both started to think that with as many years of my illness, if the diagnosis of aplastic anemia were the case, that I should be dead by now. He referred me to an appointment with a specialist at the Cross Cancer Institute in Edmonton.

In March of 2007, I had an appointment with Dr. Robert Turner in Edmonton, more blood work and another bone marrow tap. He had a diagnosis for me: I had a rare form of leukemia known as hairy cell leukemia. It is given that name because one type of white blood cells are formed with little hair-like projections on their cell surfaces. The abnormal proliferation of these hairy cells leads to reduced production of red blood cells, platelets and the other types of white cells.

Fate was with me as there were 3 chemo-therapeutic drugs known to have positive effect for treatment of hairy cell leukemia[12]. I was feeling quite ill at this time but I managed to finish classes and labs in April of 2007. Beginning of May 2007, I went to Grande Prairie hospital for 3 days of intravenous chemo, with a drug known as clanbrine.

By June, after the treatment, I noticed a big change: I no longer had the uncontrollable sleeping episodes, I no longer had to worry about falling asleep while driving. Another notable change was that for many years, I would develop a mucoid-like eye discharge; this too disappeared after the clanbrine treatment.

However, I discovered that if I was doing some hard physical labor, that I became tired quickly. Further medical investigation revealed that I had a cardiac problem, a type of left bundle branch heart block. The doctors were convinced that I had suffered a heart attack and likely had some blocked arteries.

Several trips to the cardiologists in Edmonton, angiogram studies revealed no blocked arteries. The doctors then decided that I had "idiopathic cardiomyopathy" (damage to the heart due to unknown cause). The most likely explanation is that when I was at the worst stage of the hairy cell leukemia due to a low white blood count, I developed a viral infection which damaged my heart muscle.

I was put on medication to help my heart and in 2017, I had a pacemaker installed which regulated my heartbeat and increased the heart efficiency.

Every 2 months or so, I go for a CBC and differential blood cell count, so far so good, the hairy cell leukemia has not returned! (When I had the treatment in 2007, the doctor said I would be "OK" for at least ten years.)

It is not known why some people (mostly men) develop hairy cell leukemia; one speculated cause is exposure to a group of chemicals known as organo-phosphates. At one time, a number of this group of chemicals were used extensively in the livestock industry to control a number of livestock pests such as the warble fly, lice and ticks.

I still vividly remember many fall mornings, listening to 630 CHED in the heavy Chevy driving out to pregnancy test cows with gallon jugs of Neguvon in the back of the station wagon. It was not uncommon for the lids of the gallon Neguvon jugs to be a bit loose and with the heat of the car heater, I recall the distinctive smell of the Neguvon fumes that I was breathing in…..we later learned that this chemical could be absorbed and stored in fatty tissue of the body. There are many known causes of cancer and many unknown causes, I still speculate on my exposure to the organo-phosphate chemicals as the cause of my developing the chronic hairy cell leukemia (there are documented cases of hairy cell leukemia of over 30 years in duration).

There are probably many people who would describe me as naturally rather "dopey"… slow thinker and slow talker. However due to the effects of the hairy cell leukemia, I feel I functioned as if I were in a "zombie" state at times. I used to be able to do it standing up, sitting down, or lying down (sleep that is).

As I reflect back on my health issues, although I am thankful for much of my care by the human medical profession, I wish that I had been more proactive in my dealings with the health care system. An earlier diagnosis and treatment of the hairy cell leukemia may have meant that I stayed for more years in practice at Wainwright and my kids could have been closer to their Wainwright friends.

It is said that you can't change the past, but I regret that earlier diagnosis and treatment may have meant that I would have been less grumpy to my wife, children, students and clients. Perhaps I would have done more things with my family, my students and perhaps would have been sharper in my practice days. I guess I evolved to work at a pace that I could endure. Yes, I do live with many regrets.

Since 2020, I have been on wait list status for an ankle fusion and having my 2 knees replaced, the Covid pandemic was a major disruption to the health care system but it seems to function slowly regardless.

I used to look bad, feel bad; I feel better, but the ladies say that I still look bad. Oh well.

Chapter Eight

PRACTICE REFLECTIONS

Looking back over 55 years ago, many of the early cattle cases involved vitamin A deficiency. The long winter months of western Canada dictate that cattle are fed dry hay, grain, etc. which can be very low in an essential nutrient for man and beast: vitamin A.

Vitamin A deficiency[1] can cause a host of issues: blindness, fainting spells, convulsions, poor growth rate, lowered reproductive performance, decreased resistance to infection and birth deformities to name a few. In the early 1970's, we observed many newborn calves with cleft lip, cleft palate, hydrocephalus (dome skull due to excess brain fluid) as well as blind, convulsing cattle. By the 1980's as veterinarians, we saw very few if any such cases. The new technology of injectable vitamin A allowed ranchers to prevent the deficiency problem as cows could be injected, absorb and then store a 3- month supply of vitamin A in their livers. Another advancement was the production of vitamin A powder which could be added to the daily feed of the cows or provided as part of a mineral mix for the cows.

It was a matter of educating livestock owners on the importance of providing vitamin A supplementation to their livestock and in retrospect, I think veterinarians, district agriculturists, media and extension personnel did an excellent job to get the message out. Very gratifying to go from a situation where 33 out of 46 calves on one farm were born hopelessly deformed to rarely seeing the problem at all in practice.

Another frequent problem in the early 1970's was that of the "water-belly steer". This condition, urolithiasis[2], is the congregation of minerals into a hard mass (a urolith or kidney or bladder stone). Most usually, the stones would form in the urinary bladder and in male cattle and sheep, these species have an "S" curve (the sigmoid flexure) of the penis, a stone could get caught (stuck) in the curve. A total blockage of urine flow could result, if the farmer did not notice signs of the affected animal straining, kicking at the belly, lying down, etc. the back up of urine could become so severe as to cause the urinary bladder to rupture or the urethra (urinary tube) in the penis to rupture. Net result would then be the building of free urine in the abdominal cavity (hence the term water-belly) or a build up of urine under the skin of the belly. As veterinarians, we would do operations to remove the stone, drain the abdominal cavity and suture the bladder, etc. Some of these animals suffered too much kidney damage from the back pressure of urine and would die.

(The stones would form in females but since they are anatomically superior to males having a shorter straight urethra, blockage was very rare in a female.)

In my first few years of practice in the early 1970's, shortly after a very cold spell in the fall/winter, we would be deluged with water-belly cases to deal with. Again, by the time I left practice, seeing a water-belly case was a rare occurrence. Again, progress and increased knowledge had occurred in the livestock industry. The development of automatic cattle waterers meant

PRACTICE REFLECTIONS

that the animals had 24 hour access to water, they drank more, urinated more often with less chance of minerals forming precipitate stones. No vitamin A deficiency meant that the lining of the urinary tract was healthier with less sluffing of cell masses that could serve as a nidus for mineral to aggregate on. Force feeding a bit of salt also increased the frequency of urination and lessened the chance of stone formation. We also learned that some hay species were more likely than others to cause stone formation.

In the late 1960's, early 1970's, farmers would delay castration of their male calves until the animals were yearlings (year olds); this practice was very common due to the thinking that the urethra in the penis would be larger in diameter than that of an early castrate animal. (Further studies proved that this concept was not the case, with puberty, there was really no effect for a larger urethra in the penis.)

Nonetheless, the thinking meant that in our Wainwright area, in addition to the calvings, prolapses, etc., a large portion of our veterinary work consisted of calls to castrate hundreds of yearling bulls and in the early 1970's, most of those yearling bulls also had horns to remove. These dehornings and castrations were tedious and grueling work, bloody and leaving a veterinarian with little sense of satisfaction. Growth setbacks due to pain, stress and bleeding as well as occasional post-op deaths were drawbacks to the industry.

I can comment with pride to animal welfare groups and animal rights activists, that although perfection has not been achieved in the beef industry that the improvement in regards to castration and dehorning of cattle has been immense over the past fifty plus years. Ranchers are using more polled genetics (calves are born that will not grow horns) and dehorning if necessary is performed when the calves are very young, and the horn development is not very great. Similarly most ranchers now castrate the calves as newborns before puberty has increased the size of the male organs. In cases where older cattle must be dehorned, and/or castrated, we now have available very effective drugs to alleviate pain post-operatively in cattle.

Another serious disease that was a common concern in the fifties, sixties and seventies, was coccidiosis[4,5]. Affected calves would exhibit severe bloody diarrhea, straining, convulsions, dehydration, weight loss and possible death. This disease is due to a small intracellular parasite with a complicated life cycle. One life stage of the parasite can remain dormant under the lining of the intestinal tract; most typically after a period of severe stress (cold weather) the coccidia oocysts (eggs) would burst the lining of the intestine causing severe bleeding and diarrhea.

When I first graduated from veterinary college, veterinarians prescribed sulfa drugs to treat coccidiosis, these drugs were not that effective and were basically "closing the barn door after the horse was out". However, going forward into the seventies, preventative coccidiostat drugs such as Deccox, Rumensin, amprolium, and Bovatec became available to add to the feed or water of weaned calves; the coccidiosis disease virtually was wiped off the face of the cattle industry. Overall, the cattle industry also adopted methods to reduce stress of weaned calves and our knowledge of nutrition of cattle also improved from 5 decades ago.

The exotic cattle boom of the early 1970's resulted in a lot of "wheeling and dealing" of cattle i.e. eastern Canadian cattle being shipped to western Canada, cattle sold repeatedly and moved to different areas of the country. As a result we saw the appearance and spread of diseases "new" to most western Canadian cattle: bovine virus diarrhea (BVD), ITEME (infectious thrombo-meningioencephalitis), IBR (infectious bovine rhino-tracheitis), rota virus calf scours and corona virus calf scours. At times these diseases caused devastating losses to many cattle herds in our practice area.

PRACTICE REFLECTIONS

The BVD[3] virus infects the lining of the mouth, tongue, lips, esophagus (gullet) and intestinal tract: vesicles (blisters) form which burst and leave intensely painful open ulcers. The affected animal is too sore to eat and drink, has diarrhea, dehydrates and wastes away with death following. Those that survive are usually left as chronic unhealthy "poor doers". It is a disease primarily of young weaned cattle but can affect grown cattle sometimes; the gastrointestinal signs are minor and transitory in older cattle however the virus if it infects a pregnant cow, can cause reproductive problems and birth defects depending upon the stage of pregnancy.

One of our rancher clients ran about a 600 head beef cow herd. Each fall this ranch experienced a number of death losses shortly after weaning the calves. Post mortems confirmed the presence of classical BVD lesions and we also had laboratory confirmation of BVD by the provincial Alberta Veterinary Pathology Laboratory.

At that era of time, there was a company called Pitmann-Moore which manufactured and supplied a number of pharmaceutical drugs, vaccines and medical supplies for both the human and veterinary medical fields.

One of that company's sales representatives gave Keith and I a sales pitch: the company's new technology had allowed them to create a new "live virus" vaccine for BVD: their research data showed that it was very effective in preventing BVD. Live virus technology means that a virus is modified in the lab so that its potency (virulency) to cause disease is much reduced so that when injected as a vaccine, it does survive and reproduce in the animal's body, causing vast numbers of viruses to induce the body to produce vast numbers of protective antibodies but does not cause the actual disease. The live modified (attenuated) virus vaccines are supposed to be safe and not cause any serious clinical signs. [There are killed virus vaccines, totally safe in terms of minimal clinical signs, but since they contain a set number of killed virus particles, they result in a lower number of protective antibodies produced by the body and even then, the protection does not last as long as with using a live vaccine.]

"Bedazzled" (or bewitched) by the presentation on Pitman-Moore's new BVD vaccine breakthrough (Mucovax 3 was the trade name), Dr. Leitch and I advised our client to vaccinate their calves that fall to prevent BVD losses. Our clients used the great new BVD vaccine to vaccinate their 600+ calves that fall upon our advice. Within a few days after vaccinations, there were many sick calves exhibiting all the classical lesions and signs of BVD! Final death loss was 63 calves, about five to six times the "usual" deaths due to BVD in previous years in that herd.

We phoned Pitman-Moore's head office in Kalamazoo, Michigan. After about three weeks of stonewalling, the company sent out an investigative team to visit our client's ranch. By this time there were no more active living BVD cases in the herd. The company representatives took blood samples and swabs and left without giving us any answers.

About two weeks later, they sent us a letter – tests for IBR virus, parainfluenza virus were negative but sorry they DID NOT HAVE ENOUGH BLOOD SERUM FOR BVD TESTING! Total copout as BVD was the complaint (the company took the blood samples)!

Dr. Leitch and I were left high and dry by Pitman-Moore. We worked out an arrangement with our clients whereby we provided bull evaluations, pregnancy testing and other veterinary work at no charge to compensate them for the increased calf BVD death loss after vaccination.

Science is never settled; years later researchers established the fact that if a pregnant cow was exposed to the BVD virus in the early stages of pregnancy, the developing calf embryo would come to recognize the BVD virus as part of its own body. The calf would develop as "normal", be born and survive carrying a particular strain of the BVD virus. Later on in its life, if that calf were exposed to a different strain of the BVD virus, it develops a full-blown case of BVD. We now use the term persistently infected (P.I.), for those animals. There was now an explanation for what happened in our clients' herd following the live BVD virus vaccination.

Pitman-Moore had tested their vaccine but obviously not using animals in cattle herds where there were likely P.I. animals. I ponder the recent COVID vaccination programs in human medicine and I'm worried, not for myself as I'm near the end of my run of life, but worried about the COVID vaccines that were "pushed" upon people in a panic and politically expedient manner. The pre-market testing of these COVID vaccines was too minimal for the radically new technology utilized in the manufacture of these RNA vaccines. I'm a proponent of vaccines but only effective, safe vaccines and I will relate further on this issue when I discuss parvovirus disease in dogs.

In the early seventies another frustrating disease condition we frequently saw in practice was grain overload (lactic acid poisoning[6]); this was a man-made condition caused by feeding too much grain too quickly to cattle. Sometimes cattle accidently broke into a grain bin. The main stomach of a ruminant species (such as a cow) is a huge storage vat for hay, grain and water. When a cow chews its cud, it regurgitates a portion of feed and chews the feed into smaller particles. The rumen of a healthy cow is an ecosystem of various species of bacteria and protozoa (one cell organisms) which aid in the breakdown of feed.

If a cow eats too much grain (before a gradual adaptation) there is a sudden shift in the bacterial population; a lactobacillus bacteria breaks down the starches in grain and lactic acid is a product of that bacteria's metabolism. Lactic acid is absorbed into the cow's blood stream, blood pH becomes acidic, cells are damaged by the acid, the lining of the rumen is "burned" by the acid, water from the blood stream is drawn into the rumen, leading to severe shock and dehydration result which can lead to death of the animal.

At that time in veterinary medicine, as veterinarians, we tried a number of treatments; laxatives and anti-acids by stomach tube, intravenous fluids, rumenotomy (which involved surgically opening up an incision into the rumen and manually removing the grain) as well as a procedure called rumen lavage. The rumen lavage technique involves putting a large diameter stomach tube down to the rumen, then connecting it to a water hose, running in warm water, disconnecting and then the back wash would wash out some grain. Repeating the process several times could gradually wash the grain and lactic acid out of the rumen.

We dealt with individual cases of grain overload but often we were faced with a "wreck": an entire herd of cattle affected at the same time. Near Christmas of 1985, a client had a pen of about 80 yearling heifers on hay and a self-feeder with a grain mixture. A high level of salt was added to the grain mixture to prevent the animals from eating too much at one time. Just before Christmas the client had to be away from home and a cold snap down to -30 C set in. The self-feeder ran down to empty; the feed company had been called to come out and fill up the self-feeder but due to a bad storm, the feed company was late in delivering the grain mix. Inadvertently someone at the feed mill forgot to add the restricting salt to the grain mixture.

Everything was wrong in the situation: the heifers were very hungry, the cold weather induced a 30 to 40% increase in energy demand for them to stay warm and the kicker was the missing high salt level in the grain mixture.

I got called out to the client's farm on December 24, there were several heifers down and unable to stand up; there was no doubt the diagnosis was grain overload by the signs shown by the heifers and the history of the circumstances.

PRACTICE REFLECTIONS

The client enlisted the help of some neighbors and they dragged the down heifers into a horse trailer, hauled them to our clinic. With the help of our associate veterinarian, Dr. Peder Paulsen, I started these animals on the rumen lavage treatment, put in intravenous catheters and hooked each up to five-gallon jugs of intravenous fluids. So much for Christmas eve! I had a brief time at home with Eileen and the kids for the opening of presents while Dr. Paulsen (who was single) kept I.V.'s going, etc.

Christmas day had the client hauling in more sick animals and we spent the day treating and then hauling out the ones that did not survive. Our success rate with our treatments was much poorer than with other cases in the past; I think the -30 C weather exposure added significantly to the shock these animals suffered. Overall, there were 26 deaths out of the 80 heifers in spite of all of our efforts. The feed company reached some sort of settlement with the client. Overall, it was not a very merry Christmas that year for all concerned!

Another major disease issue we dealt with was calf scours (basically the shits), (diarrhea and dehydration and often death). There are many causes of calf scours such as E-coli bacteria[7] salmonella bacteria, rotoviruses, coronaviruses and intra-cellular parasites: cryptosporidiosis and coccidiosis. Many management practices and stress due to inclement weather are also involved in the scours complex.

In most of our farm animal species such as cattle, it is absolutely critical that their newborn nurse an adequate amount of the first milk (colostrum) within the first few hours after being born. Colostrum contains protective antibodies (gamma globulins) which provide the newborn protection to any infectious disease agents which the mother has been exposed to during her life. Without the colostral antibodies, a newborn calf is susceptible to one disease after another; they do poorly and in spite of a lot of treatments, they most often go on to die. (Human pediatric medicine is much easier as the human placenta allows for antibodies to enter the baby during pregnancy; animals have different types of placenta than humans and in-utero passage of antibodies cannot occur in horses, cattle, sheep and pigs.

So along with dealing with calving, foaling, lambing and farrowing problems, veterinary medicine in the spring months, veterinarians were treating literally hundreds of scouring calves, foals, piglets and lambs. In the early years we treated these cases with antibiotics, oral and intravenous fluids. Again, the exotic cattle boom led to a lot of sales and mixing of cattle, a perfect way to transfer disease agents from one herd to another.

In the early 1970's, in our practice, we tied the scouring calf down on a table and threaded a two-inch needle down the jugular vein to hook up to the intravenous fluids. Very frustrating for if the calf struggled, the needle could come out of the vein; the intravenous fluid would then run OTF (on the floor) or under the calf's skin.

A very great advance was when we learned about human medicine intravenous catheters (long flexible tubes that could be threaded down a calf's jugular vein). The calf could be placed in a small pen while its intravenous fluids ran in and the calf could have freedom of movement during treatment! Little worry of a needle getting moved out of the vein! I.V. catheters were a great boom to both small and large animal veterinary medicine.

Another advancement in the treatment of the scouring calves, was the advent of the esophageal tube feeder. Originally this was a solid stainless steel rod with a bit of a bulb on one end. The idea of the bulb was that it would not go through the larynx into the trachea (windpipe) and one could feel the bulb under the skin of the calf's neck if it was correctly placed in the gullet (esophagus) to the calf's stomach to administer fluids orally. We did give oral fluids by stomach tube and tried to teach our clients how to pass a stomach tube, however, people make errors and sometimes fluids wound up in the lungs if the tube got inadvertently placed in the windpipe. The esophageal feeder was much more fool proof in that regard however, we did see some severe problems with its use; rough use resulted in a lever-like action and rupture of the esophagus of a calf. Newer esophageal feeders are now made out of softer, more flexible plastic material.

In those early years, we made the intravenous fluid by adding baking soda (sodium bicarbonate) and white table salt to water. This was a crude way of replenishing the electrolytes lost due to the diarrhea.

Further research led to the development of very good balanced electrolyte solutions and powders for the treatment of dehydrated calves. The oral powders can be mixed with water and given by the owners; many scouring calves are successfully treated at home before severe shock and dehydration set in, eliminating the need for veterinary intravenous treatment.

Another learning curve for our veterinary treatment of scouring calves concerned the use , overuse and abuse of antibiotic treatments for scouring calves. In the early 70's, we knew that E.coli and sometimes salmonella bacteria could be the causes of calf scours. If 3 or 4 days treatment with a particular antibiotic failed to cure a calf, we switched to another antibiotic and sometimes yet another. In time, we learned that this practice "knocked out" all of the good bacteria species in the calf's intestine and was counter-productive to curing the scours. Over the course of a few years, veterinary medicine established that intravenous and/or oral fluids and electrolytes were most important in treatment of the scouring calves.

The veterinary clinic at Wainwright had an isolation area; its main use was for hospitalization of the scouring calf cases. As the cattle boom of the early 70's went on, Dr. Leitch and I made the decision to add on to our existing clinic, so that we had 3 calving/Caesarean headgate areas. We also had a separate building constructed to allow more isolation pens and a post-mortem room separate from the main clinic building. It seemed like a good decision at the time but when the bottom fell out of cattle prices in 1974/75, it was financially a great burden for us. I often envied human medical doctors who could work out of a taxpayer funded hospital!

Over the course of the 1970's, there was the development of calf scour vaccines to prevent the development of this disease. Our practice had two clients who participated in Dr. Steve Acres' piliform vaccine field trials for E.coli scours; this new vaccine was designed to be given to pregnant cows, thus stimulating the production of protective antibodies to the pili of the E.coli bacteria and these antibodies were then secreted into the colostrum of the cows. Over the years, other advances were the development of vaccines for rotavirus calf scours, coronavirus calf scours and a clostridial vaccine for another specific type of calf scours.

The cattle industry also learned a lot about the role of clean calving grounds, shelter, good nutrition and reducing stress as ways to prevent calf scours. Calf scours is still a problem in some herds today, but we have advanced markedly from my early days in practice when there were herds of cattle that experienced over a 50% death loss due to scours.

Baby pig diarrhea (scours) was also a common disease issue for hog producers, again there was progress in vaccine development for the hog industry. Although the bulk of our practice dealt with cattle, we did have a number of large hog producers in the Wainwright practice area. I recall one time a hog producer started to experience a severe outbreak of baby pig scours and severe death loss of piglets. As we visited his farm, we discovered a rather unusual cause for the problem; the source of water for the mother sows was a dugout with a filter in the water line from the dugout to the hog barn. The owner removed the old filter but forgot to replace it; the water line plugged off so no water was going to the waterers in the hog barn. Paradoxically, the sows "knew" that there was no water and they just laid down and made no attempt to try to drink. Without water, the sows' milk production went down to zero, the piglets were starving and eating manure leading to the development of scours, dehydration and death. The producer did not have a mysterious new type of baby pig scours in his herd, a lesson in management and husbandry was learned in a hard way.

Another huge change in veterinary medicine from my early days in practice, was growth of equine horse practice to what it is today. I can recall giving a horse owner a quote of $100.00 for work on his horse: "forget it" he said, "I'll just ship him and start another colt I have". Today, I am amazed and gratified by the number of equine practitioners and what level of expense horse owners are willing to pay in today's world. Again, the advancements in equine medicine have been huge; I recall being told as a veterinary student about the Roberts' treatment for a "bleeder" (horse that suffers severe nosebleed); this treatment was injection of formaldehyde into the jugular vein of the affected horse! Happy to say that equine medicine has progressed from some very barbaric treatments and practices!

We sometimes saw cases of tetanus[8] in horses. Horses and people are very susceptible to developing tetanus which can often be fatal in spite of exhaustive treatment. The condition is easily prevented by vaccination of horses and people with tetanus toxoid. The tetanus bacteria can grow in deep wounds; the bacteria produces a toxin (poison) which affects the nervous system causing paralysis and death. Tetanus toxoid is a vaccine containing a small amount of the toxin which stimulates the body to produce protective antibodies to the tetanus toxin. Vaccination for tetanus is a "must" for horse owners.

There are successes in veterinary medicine but also frustrations; a disease called equine infectious anemia (swamp fever) caused by a virus causes loss of a number of horses each year in Canada. To date, researchers have been unsuccessful in producing an effective vaccine for this disease.

A disease of horses and humans that can be a problem is Western Equine Encephalomyelitis (WEE), (sleeping sickness[9]). The causative agent in a virus which can be spread by mosquitoes and wildlife such as water bird species can serve as reservoirs for the WEE virus. The incidence of this disease was usually increased in wet years in which there were high mosquito numbers. Paradoxically in the Wainwright practice area, most cases of WEE occurred in August and September (drier months), presumably due to the build-up of the virus in wild water fowl which lead to mosquito larvae being infected while in the water stage of development.

The clinical cases of WEE could vary from relatively mild to severe convulsions and death. I recall the sad experience of one client who had 5 horses with WEE, in spite of supportive care at our clinic, all went on to progress to severe convulsions, necessitating euthanasia for humane reasons. It was devastating to present five empty halters back to five kids who lost their riding horses.

Some horses would experience milder signs of WEE; stupor or sleep like state, inactivity, in-appetite, constipation, etc. With supportive case, these horses would recover enough to be mobile, eat and drink and function in life. However, most had loss of training due to the viruses' damage to the brain.

I recall one case – an Appaloosa mare, submitted to our clinic; I hospitalized her for a few days. On weekends when I went back to the clinic, I brought our four-year old daughter, Kerry with me and while I was doing treatments, I hoisted Kerry on to the back of this horse where Kerry sat for "hours". The mare made a recovery to the state of back to eating, defecating, etc. and when the owner came to pick her up, I made the comment "what a nice horse she was when I let Kerry sit on her back".

"What"! the owner exclaimed, "she has bucked off everyone who has tried to ride her, I only keep that bleep-bleep horse because she's my wife's pet"! Obviously, the WEE virus had "numbed" her brain so that she was a quiet horse for Kerry!

When I was still a student at veterinary college, there was a researcher at the Fulton Lab who was conducting research into the WEE virus for vaccine development. At that era of time, researchers would replicate the WEE virus in embryonating chicken eggs. The eggs would be cracked open, a slurry of the contents would be prepared and then some of the slurry would be aspirated with a mouth pipette so that the slurry with high numbers of the virus could be used for processing to produce a vaccine. One day, she had a "whoops" and aspirated some of the slurry into her mouth; she related to me that she did develop a mild case of WEE, headaches for a time, fever, drowsiness, etc. but recovered.

In 1977, I had a 2800 pound Simmental bull kick me in the side of my right knee, rupturing the cruciate ligaments in the knee joint. I had surgery in the Misercordia Hospital to repair the ligaments and a heavy plaster support cast was put on my leg. The man in the other hospital bed had a brace under his left arm, a connecting rod (with an adjustable tension knob) linked to another circular brace around his chest. He relayed to me that in the previous year, he had contacted the sleeping sickness virus and went into such severe convulsions that before medical help arrived, he had fractured his left shoulder blade and arm due to the flailing of the severe convulsions. For over a month he was in a coma, when he came to it took six weeks before he could recognize his wife and family. (His arm had healed but he could not lift it very high up.) The purpose of the braces and support rod were to gradually "push" his arm up higher. WEE had serious lasting effects on him.

Going into the 1980's a new disease, West Nile, appeared in Canada; also due to a virus which can affect the brain of both horses and humans.

There are safe, effective vaccines for horses for WEE (and the Eastern, Venezuelan and Japanese forms of the virus) as well as for West Nile; I strongly advise all horse owners in western Canada to vaccinate their horses in the spring of the year for sleeping sickness and West Nile! (And for humans, do your best to ward off the carrier of those viruses – the pesky mosquito.)

Again, reflecting back to my first years of veterinary practice, a virus disease known as canine distemper[10] was relatively common. It could be devastating especially for young puppies. I recall a client who had a litter of 10 German Shorthair Pointer puppies; from some unknown source, the canine distemper virus affected all 10 puppies, in spite of supportive care, 6 of the 10 died. The survivors were left with "mottled teeth" (due to high fever at the time of enamel development); 3 of the four survivors developed a nervous "tic" of a front leg and they were not very healthy as they matured. There were vaccines for canine distemper and we preached as much as we could that dog owners should vaccinate their dogs to prevent this disease. I think our campaign was successful as I remember a 12-year gap before I observed another case of canine distemper in a rescue dog.

There is a saying that Mother Nature abhors a vacuum; an observation over the years for both human and veterinary medicine is that while we may "solve" one disease problem, another new one appears.

As veterinarians, just as we were "celebrating" the control of canine distemper and canine hepatitis in mid 70's, a new and utterly devastating disease of dogs appeared: parvovirus[16]. This disease caused severe bloody stinky diarrhea followed by severe

PRACTICE REFLECTIONS

dehydration and death. It was a new virus disease (and being a virus, it was not sensitive to antibiotics). In young puppies, the parvovirus could cause inflammation of the heart muscle and death. Our best efforts were those of supportive fluids given intravenously and other supportive drugs in the hope that the dog's body would eventually fight off the virus.

In those days, there were no effective canine parvovirus vaccines. Research had established that parvovirus of dogs was similar to the mink enteritis virus; some veterinarians in desperation vaccinated clients' dogs with mink enteritis vaccine. It did not work! At some point, a veterinarian in Alberta heard about a new wonderful parvovirus vaccine made in the U.S.A. by a company called Corn Husker. This veterinarian made a trip to the U.S.A. and smuggled a rather large quantity of the Corn Husker parvovirus vaccine into Canada. No doubt he did well with his parvovirus vaccination clinics but alas the vaccine was no more effective than urinating on a dog's left hindleg!

Fortunately, in about 2 years, a safe, effective vaccine for parvovirus was developed....I recommend it as a must for all dog owners.

Back in time, the 1950's, as a young boy of 5 or 6 years old, I recall Dad's cattle would develop "bumps" on their backs as spring approached. These bumps were due to a parasite, the warble grub[17], which had a rather complicated life cycle. In the summer months, the adult female warble fly would zoom around cattle, landing to deposit her eggs on the hair of the legs and lower body of a cow. The fly's activity would annoy and make a cow nervous; she would take off running with her tail virtually straight up in the air and run into a slough of water to gain some relief from the irritation of the warble fly. (This behavior was known as "gadding about".)

When a cow licked her haircoat, she would ingest the eggs/larvae of the warble fly; these newly hatched larvae (grubs) would burrow into the lining of the mouth, then into deeper tissues of a cow's body all the while munching on the cow's flesh as these grubs grew in size. As spring approached, the grubs (larvae) would make their way up through the muscles of the cow's back, then under the skin of the cow's back where the grubs would chew out a breathing hole in the cow's hide (skin). Upon the event of warmer weather, the grub would chew its way out, fall to the ground, pupate into an adult warble fly and its life cycle repeat again.

This parasite caused severe economic damage for the cattle industry: lowered milk production, lowered weight gains, lowered feed efficiency, damaged meat and damaged hides. All provinces of Canada established Warble Control zones; cattle producers were required to treat their cattle for warbles. There were inspections on farms, at auction markets and slaughter houses. Any evidence of warble grubs meant that farmer's location was traced and mandatory treatments were charged to the farmer.

In the early years of this control program, a chemical, rotenone, was mixed with warm water and brushed onto cattle's backs in the spring. The rotenone chemical would enter the grub's breathing hole, go through the grub's cuticle and cause paralysis and death of the grub. The idea of this treatment was to break the life cycle of the warble fly but it was somewhat akin to closing the barn door after the horse ran out: the grubs had feasted all winter in the cattle's bodies.

One spring, before Dad had treated the cattle for the warble grubs, my brothers and I discovered that if one applied careful thumb and finger pressure, it was possible to "pop" a live grub out of its breathing hole in the cow's hide. We would put a few of these live grubs (which wiggled and squirmed) in one's pants pocket before going to school. The next step was to drop one or two of these live grubs down the back of the dress of the girl sitting ahead of oneself. There is a girl called Sally who would probably shoot me on site if she met up with me today!

Later on in time, a number of pour-on organo-phosphate chemicals became available, these drugs could be poured on the skin of a cow's back, be absorbed through the skin and then into the cow's body tissues. When warble grubs ate the cow's tissue, the grubs would get a dose of the drug which killed the grubs in the fall of the year before they could feast all winter in the bodies of cattle. The cattle industry suffered far less damaged meat and hides. The organo-phosphate drugs were effective but overdoses could occur, treatment at the wrong time of the year could present problems and sometimes accidental spillage on a human's skin could cause nasty problems. These chemicals are stored in fatty tissue so adherence to withdrawal times was a must. In addition, milking dairy cows could not be treated with these drugs as residues in milk would occur.

One fall, I was out pregnancy testing a herd of Charolais cows and the owner's wife had the task of applying the pour-on, Neguvon, on the backs of the pregnant cows to treat for warbles. The Neguvon was supplied in one-gallon jugs; on the farm the standard procedure was to pour some of the Neguvon liquid in a pail and then dip a measuring dipper in the pail to get the required dose per cow. The wife had placed an ice cream pail with the Neguvon on a cross brace which ran across the chute. A somewhat wild cow threw her head up, breaking the cross brace and the ice cream pail with the Neguvon landed and spilled on the wife's head.

She ran to the house and had a long shower. However, some Neguvon had been absorbed through her skin. She related that for two years afterward she experienced headaches and nervous problems (again Neguvon is stored in body fat).

A significant improvement was the discovery of a drug called ivermectin, it was very effective and much safer than the organo-phosphate. To its credit, the original pharmaceutical company to patent ivermectin, has provided free ivermectin to many third world countries, virtually eliminating most internal parasites in children of those countries. (As an aside, ivermectin has some effects on the immune system and has been touted as an aid in the treatment of Covid-19 and some forms of cancer in humans.)

The warble control program was very successful, again I can recall many years in practice where I no longer observed any positive cases of warble infestation.

One day in the spring of 1970, an elderly rancher from the Czar area arrived at the clinic with a calving cow. The head of the calf was protruding from the cow's vulva; in technical terms, the birth presentation was that of anterior with bilateral carpal flexion, that is the front legs were bent underneath it's body, rendering birth impossible. The rancher was not sure how long the cow had been trying to calve until he had located her on a large pasture. Since the carotid arteries pump blood into the head region at higher blood pressure, due to pressure of the cow's vagina on the neck region of the calf blood fluid (due to lower venous blood pressure) becomes retained. As a result, the head of the calf was very swollen, and the tongue of the calf was extremely swollen!

I administered an epidural (spinal) nerve block to reduce the cow's straining. With the aid of a bit of lubricant, I was able to push the calf's head back into the cow's uterus. This allowed room for me to straighten out the front legs of the calf and then bring the head back into a normal birth presentation and position (i.e. head on top of the two front legs).

When I delivered the calf, it had a heartbeat but would not breathe. (In cases of prolonged labor, the placental attachments to the wall of the uterus start to separate. This results in reduced oxygen and nutrients to the calf, decreasing the vitality of the calf or even its death.)

Frantically I tried several little "tricks" to stimulate its respiration, including intravenous injection of a respiratory stimulant drug. I also tried manual compression/decompression of the calf's chest. I spent a considerable amount of time trying to resuscitate the calf to no avail and its heartbeat stopped.

As I knelt in utter dejection in front of the dead calf, the old rancher offered these words of advice: "Boy", he said, "you have to remember that you can never save them all". I think those words helped me get through many situations where I lost a patient.

On a side note, for the 1971 calving season, we got a medical grade oxygen tank equipped with air hose, Venturi valve to a plastic face mask. Indeed, over the following years, we felt that we saved a fair number of "unresponsive" calves by administration of oxygen as well as the respiratory stimulant.

For many of my early years of veterinary practice, a frequent case presentation would be that of retained placenta; the placenta or afterbirth is not passed as it normally should be after the birth of the offspring has occurred. Decomposition of the retained placenta by a variety of bacterial species in essence causes the placental tissues to rot (the smell is very atrocious). Absorption of various bacterial toxins may cause the affected cow to become very ill, even though the uterus may resist the passage of bacteria to the rest of the body.

We were taught in veterinary college that for the bovine (cattle) species, if the placenta was not passed in 48 hours, that manual removal was required. For many years in veterinary practice, veterinarians spent hours and hours with one hand and arm inside a cow breaking down the placental attachments to the uterine wall. We also gave antibiotics to the cow and placed anti-microbial boluses in the uterus. In the process, we invariably acquired the rotten stench!

Further research established the fact that in most cases of retained placenta in the cow, manual removal caused damage to the uterus which could affect the future fertility of the cow. Today, the general consensus is to cover with antibiotics and let the placenta in essence rot out on its own. Some things in veterinary medicine have evolved greatly.

The equine species is much different than cattle for retained placenta in a mare is regarded as an emergency if the placenta is not passed within six hours or so after foaling. Oxytocin, antibiotics, other drugs and manual removal are the norm for retained placenta in a mare to prevent her death or the development of founder (laminitis).

The causes of retained placenta are varied but nutritional factors can go a long way in the prevention of retained placenta. It was learned that adequate levels of the mineral selenium and vitamins A and E would greatly reduce the incidence of retained placenta in cattle. What was a rather common case for veterinarians (i.e. retained placenta in a cow) became fairly rare as the message on nutrition was adopted by more and more farmers and ranchers!

In veterinary medicine there have been phases of time when various procedures or treatments have been the current "fads". I think that the same holds true for human medicine. When our kids were young in the 1970's, colds (respiratory illness) were very common in young kids. Eileen and other mothers would take crying, miserable, snot-nosed and coughing kids to the medical clinic where the medical doctors would prescribe antibiotics such as the newer semi-synthetic penicillins; penbritin and amoxicillin. In light of the fact that most of the respiratory illnesses were likely due to a virus this practice was questionable as most all viruses are not affected by antibiotics. Perhaps the medical doctors prescribed those prescriptions to keep the "crazy" mothers out of their office? In all fairness, perhaps the antibiotics prevented secondary bacterial complications.

Once there was a pharmaceutical company, Burroughs Wellcome which made a number of drugs for both human and veterinary medicine. The company's logo or symbol was that of a horse inside of a circle; this logo was featured on all of their products. Again, in the 1970's, they started to market a newly licensed antibiotic, trimethoprim, in combination with a sulfa drug. There was a liquid form for oral use marketed under one brand name for human use and under another brand name for veterinary use. (The ingredients were essentially the same.)

Our daughter, Kerry, was in kindergarten at that time and one of the local medical doctors, Dr. Flynn, had prescribed the human trimethoprim product to treat Kerry when she had a cold. Mrs. Flynn, the doctor's wife, was Kerry's kindergarten teacher at that time. Later in the winter when Kerry had another cold, I had noticed that her previous prescription was actually the same as the veterinary product…..I used that to treat Kerry. Later in "show and tell" at kindergarten, Kerry proudly announced to the class "my Daddy gives me horse medicine" (i.e. symbol on the bottle).

Mrs. Flynn told her husband Dr. Flynn, and I later had to face his rather embarrassing quizzing at a social function in Wainwright!

As I reflect back again on my early years of practice, it is somewhat gratifying to think that perhaps I and my contemporaries laid some of the "groundwork" for the current state of veterinary practice. It was one thing for us to encourage vaccination of dogs and cats, but it was another thing to suggest to rather bemused clients that their dog required teeth cleaning. Indeed, in our practice in the early 1970's, if we convinced a couple clients per year to have their pets' teeth cleaned, that was about it. Today veterinary dentistry is a large part of most veterinary practices and indeed there are now veterinarians and veterinary technicians who specialize in veterinary dentistry!

At times life seems like a series of trial and error, certainly the same may be said of both human and veterinary medicine. During the 1970's, 1980's and into the 1990's, there were a number of pharmaceutical products of the nitrofuran chemical group. These compounds were used to combat bacterial infections, etc. in the forms of topical skin/wound ointments, sprays, pills (boluses) and oral liquids. In veterinary medicine we used them extensively for treatments of wire cuts of horses, E.colibacillosis (scours) of calves, lambs, baby piglets, and urinary tract and respiratory infections. We used those compounds without protection such as wearing gloves.

Although these products were tested before licensing in Canada and the U.S.A., with the passage of time, they became suspected of being carcinogenic (cancer causing) and mutagenic (causing genetic changes). In human medicine, nitrofuran compounds were commonly used to treat cystitis (bladder infection) and other infections. Another problem with nitrofuran usage became recognized in human medicine: the induction of irreversible interstitial pulmonary fibrosis (in essence rigid scar tissue formation in the walls of the alveoli i.e. air sacs of the lungs). I mention this on a personal basis, a friend and colleague, Dr. Jim Henderson, was at one time treated with nitrofurans and indeed later in his life developed interstitial pulmonary fibrosis, eventually the cause of his death. As I mentioned before, many things have been learned the hard way in both human and veterinary medicine.

PRACTICE REFLECTIONS

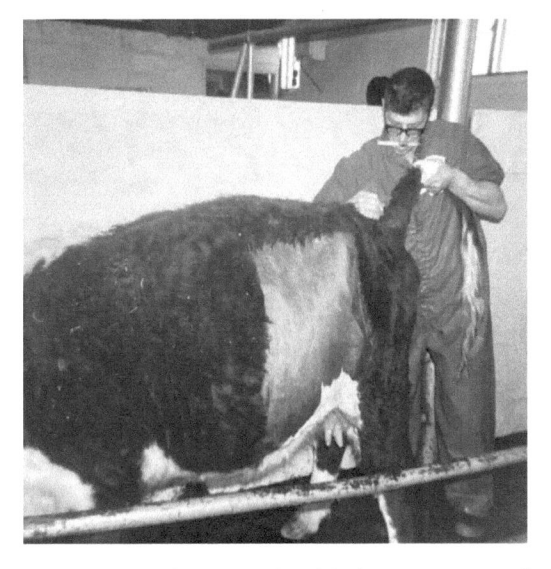

Administering an epidural nerve block before cesarean on a heifer

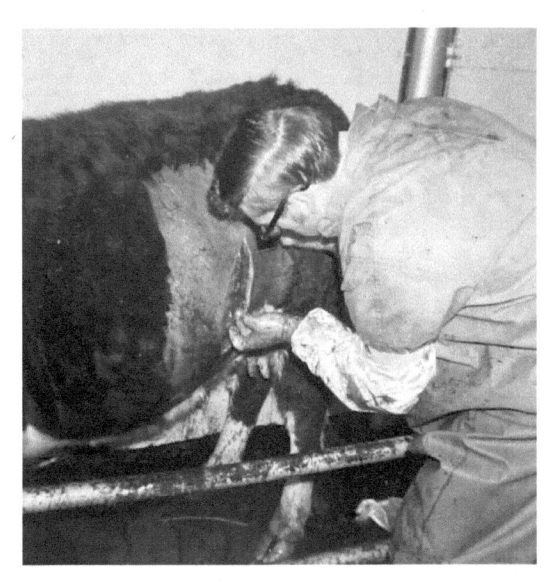

Suturing up cesarean incision

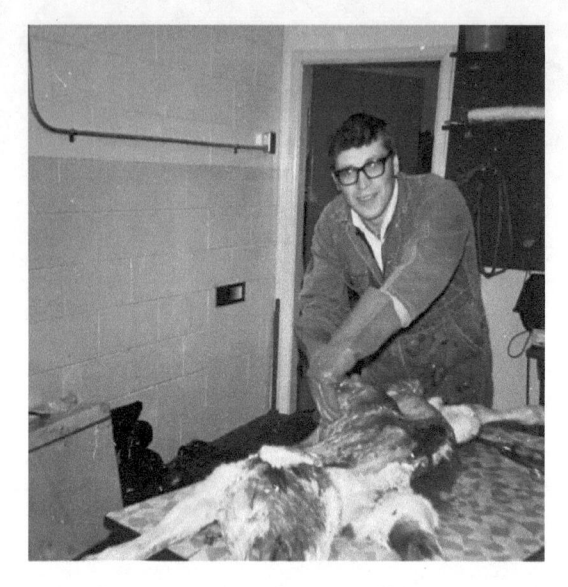

Post-mortem on a calf

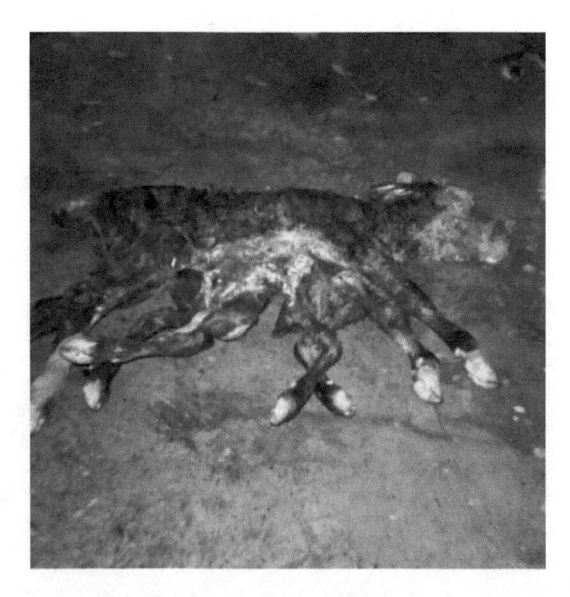

Eight-legged calf: body of one twin absorbed into body of the first twin.

Chapter Nine

GUTS, GORE AND MORE

Post-mortems or autopsies were a large part of veterinary practice; to prove a cause of an animal's death or to determine the cause of an animal's death. Performing post-mortems yielded a vast body of knowledge as to the lesions and mechanisms of disease. However, as in human medicine, in veterinary medicine, we sometimes cannot determine a cause of death, even upon doing a post-mortem.

I can recall a number of years that were the "animal mutilation years" and "aliens mutilating animals". As usual, the media was able to stoke the claims that people or aliens or cults were killing cattle, sheep and cutting off the external genitalia, tongues, etc. It is a fact that ruminant species such as cattle and sheep when they die, their bodies' decomposition is rapid and very marked (especially in hot weather) leading to bloating of the carcass. The severe internal pressures caused by gases of decomposition cause protrusion of the tongue, swelling and bulging out of the rectum and genitalia. For predators and scavengers (coyotes, bear, ravens, magpies, etc. the bulging out tissues are the first parts of the carcass that they will eat.

I recall one case, a dead Hereford steer and it appeared as if someone had neatly cut out the skin of the area of the prepuce and sheath of the urinary/penis opening in the form of a neat circle. However, when I skinned back the skin surrounding this neat circle, very obvious tooth marks were evident in the skin! Upon opening the carcass further, the steer had extensive lesions of a chronic pneumonia (the most likely cause of death). No alien or cult influence, but somehow the owners would refuse to believe the cause of death was not deliberate killing and mutilating!

While the calls for veterinarians to investigate the mutilation deaths created some work for veterinary practice, it seemed like most of those calls occurred on weekends, holidays and evenings.

A lot of our post-mortem calls would involve going out to a farm to a dead cow or horse, however, our practice had a post-mortem room and we were able to convince many livestock owners to load and haul dead animals and bring the carcasses to our clinic for post-mortem.

I recall many nights, at 1:00 a.m. in the morning (after dealing with a day's work of calvings, prolapses, sick calves, scouring calves, etc.) having a pile of dead calves to post-mortem before I could go home for the day. Often, we would have samples to submit to the Veterinary Diagnostic Pathology Lab in Edmonton. The "fresher" the samples, the greater the chances of getting an accurate lab diagnosis…..samples had to go out on the bus at 8:00 a.m. the next morning!

Our clinic had an arrangement with the town of Wainwright whereby the town landfill would always have a trench ditch for us to dump the post-mortem remains for burial disposal. We had to haul these remains out to the town landfill so at one point our clinic had an old red Chev pick-up. We employed young high school students to clean at our clinic, assist where required and haul out the "deads".

I recall a time when we started to get comments and phone calls to the effect that we didn't need to advertise our mistakes. Then we learned that our young employee on his way to the town landfill (with the back of the truck box full of dead, stinky carcasses) was taking the main street route on his way to the landfill. He enjoyed the gasping, gagging people as he drove down main street. We had a good discussion with him as to a more appropriate route to the landfill!

The last part of the route to the landfill involved crossing over the main CN railway track: at that time a young girl was the "gut truck" driver and as she sped over the railway track, a dead cow carcass fell onto the tracks! I turned grey very early in my life!

Crazy stuff happens: one Sunday I had a farmer phone me about one of his calves that died suddenly. I was about to leave on a country call to a uterine prolapse case so I suggested to the farmer that he bring in the dead calf and just leave it outside the door to our post-mortem room, I would take it in when I got back from my country call. I had more calls that Sunday and I forgot about the dead calf. Next morning, I did remember and when I opened the post-mortem door, to my dismay, a town dog had performed the post-mortem! Most of the carcass was eaten, there was literally nothing left to form a diagnosis upon. It was a very difficult and embarrassing conversation that I had to make with the owner! More grey hair!

As I mentioned previously, in regards to rabies, doing post-mortems put veterinarians at constant risk of contracting a zoonotic disease (i.e. transmissible from animal to human). Once I performed a post-mortem on a dead sow and submitted samples to the diagnostic lab. Several days later, the lab notified me of a positive culture of a species of salmonella bacteria (one species of note caused in the course of history severe death losses of humans due to typhoid fever). At about this time, one of our young employees (who had hauled out the sow's carcass) started to experience severe vomiting and diarrhea. In a couple of days, his older brother (who did not work at our vet clinic) also had vomiting and diarrhea. Public health authorities determined that they had contacted salmonella; the same strain as was isolated from the dead sow! The importance of wearing protective gloves and other protection and following rigid sanitation precautions can never be overstated. Our salmonella case was the subject of an article in the Canadian Journal of Medicine.

Time is of the essence and no more so when it comes to post-mortem. With warm temperature and increased time to the post-mortem, decomposition of the carcass can cause tissues to liquify, fill with gas and become extremely putrid (stinky) rendering observing meaningful lesions and making lab tests impossible.

Once I had a call from a farmer who had gone out to his pasture and found 15 dead cows. He had already called a rendering company to pick up the dead cows and when he phoned me the carcasses were already loaded in the rendering truck. This particular farmer had a well known affinity for beer; that was very evident during his phone call but he was very adamant that I come out, meet the rendering truck and do post-mortems. Against my better judgement, I went out on the call and to my worst fear, the carcasses were swollen up like hot air balloons. The putrid smell was also very high! Amidst a few zillion flies, I opened a couple of carcasses, everything was totally rotten. The best I could do was to take some samples of "soup" for testing for lead and a few other toxins. The owner was "pissed" that I could not give him a diagnosis (then again, he really was actually pissed!). Years later he managed to get himself banned from the Viking bar for 99 years!

After I left practice and was employed as an instructor at Fairview College, I still was involved with a number of post-mortems. For many years there was a Regional Diagnostic

Veterinary Pathology laboratory in Fairview. I taught a pathology course to the Animal Health Technology students and there was an arrangement to take the students to that lab, show the postmortem procedures, sampling, etc.

For many years, Dr. Bill Nagge was Head of the Pathology Lab in Fairview. He told me the story of a farmer who had sick chickens in his farm flock. Dr. Nagge asked the farmer to bring in some sick chickens to the lab; the farmer decided to shoot the sick chickens and brought them in dead to the lab. Perhaps the devil made him do it. Dr. Nagge gave the owner the diagnosis that the chickens had died of lead poisoning! (He had an actual diagnosis for the sick chickens which he reported to the farmer later on.)

Chapter Ten

PROLAPSES

In veterinary practice, we dealt with many prolapse cases; rectal prolapses, vaginal prolapses and uterine prolapses. One analogy of a prolapse is that of a stocking getting pulled in on itself.

Rectal prolapses most often occur in animals with severe diarrhea such as with the disease coccidiosis. Once the rectum has prolapsed, it is subject to trauma, perhaps freezing and sometimes predators such as coyotes, ravens, etc. While not a dire emergency, it is best if the prolapsed rectum can be replaced as soon as possible; a purse-string (tightening) suture placed around the anal sphincter and corrective measures given for the cause of the straining.

Vaginal/Cervical prolapses are most common in the bovine species but may sometimes occur in most all species. In cattle, vaginal prolapses may occur before or after a cow has calved. There is a genetic predisposition in some lines of cattle breeding, trauma at the time of breeding or assistance at the calving is sometimes a cause and vaginal/urinary infections may contribute to severe straining and the cow prolapsing the vagina. Again, while not a dire emergency, from an animal welfare standpoint, the vaginal prolapse cases should have corrective treatment soon. Spinal anesthesia (epidural) eliminates pain and straining, the prolapse is washed up and replaced. A number of different types of pins and/or sutures are then placed around the vulva to prevent the prolapse from reoccurring. Sometimes a long- acting type of spinal is employed to lessen straining after replacement.

A uterine prolapse almost always occurs within minutes to the first few hours after an animal has given birth. As the name implies, a uterine prolapse is all of the animal's uterus prolapsing out of the vagina. It is regarded as an emergency; most veterinarians prefer to go out to the farm to deal with these cases. Severe internal or external bleeding can occur; the prolapse can get caught on brush, fences, etc. and get torn, the tissue can get frozen or severely contaminated. I have observed a couple cases where the affected cows took off running and all of the uterus ripped off! I also remember several cases where the farmer did not phone the clinic, just loaded his uterine prolapse cow in a truck or horse trailer; upon arrival at the clinic, the cow would be dead in a large puddle of her own blood! The excitement of being loaded, falling down in the truck or trailer resulted in the uterus being torn and fatal bleeding occurring. Sometimes a uterine prolapse can be "massive" as there may also be intestines inside of the prolapsed uterus.

For many years in western Canada, because there were few veterinarians, many farmers and ranchers developed a "culture" of doing their own veterinary work. There were those who tried their hands at replacing vaginal prolapses. They had no means of doing spinal anesthesia so "pushing" in a vaginal prolapse was a matter of brute force (certainly very painful for the cow). After that, in addition to suturing across the vagina to keep the prolapsed vagina in, a lot of ingenuity was employed. One farmer

PROLAPSES

technique was an empty whisky bottle, a broom handle was placed down the neck of the bottle which was then placed in the cow's vagina. The exposed portion of the broom handle (sticking out of the cow's vagina) had a strap or rope wrapped around it, and the ends were brought forward to wrap around the cow's neck. When the cow strained, this contraption kept the whisky bottle and the prolapse in place! Another old-time technique was to place a rather large rock in the cow's vagina to "weigh down" the prolapse and stitches were applied across the cow's vulva.

Our practice employed at least one senior veterinary student each summer. I recall one incident, a guy brought in a Hereford cow; he had replaced a prolapsed vagina and sutured across the vulva with baler twine but she was constantly straining. He had arrived at the clinic just at noon so that had the hair on the back of my neck "bristling up" as I was booked for a country call at 1:00 p.m. As I applied a spinal, the farmer said "I'm going downtown for lunch, be back later for her".

Since this obviously had been an ongoing case for days, that left me in a bit of a foul mood, I normally would have been talking and explaining things more to the veterinary student. I cut away the farmer's baler twine and reached into the cow's vagina and felt some sort of foreign lump that was somewhat soft. The farmer had balled up a large cloth and placed that into the cow's vagina after he had pushed in the prolapse. I scooped out this lump (not talking) and let it fall on the clinic floor. Due to pressure and being wedged in the cow's vagina, it was very bloody and rather heart shaped. "Oh my God", screamed the veterinary student, "its her heart"!

At that time in veterinary practice, to alleviate post-prolapse straining by a cow, we would do a "gutsy": an alcohol spinal. A small amount of isopropyl alcohol (instead of lidocaine) would be injected into the spinal canal. The alcohol would "demyelinate" nerve fibers in the spinal cord, the net result being analogous to removing the insulation of an electric cord. The short-circuiting of the nerves would stop pain in the pelvic/vaginal area and, also stop the severe straining until tissue of the prolapse had time to heal. However, if one misjudged the amount of alcohol injected, there was a risk of paralyzing the nerves to the hind legs!

Many years later when I was an instructor at Fairview College, while discussing prolapses with the Animal Health Technology students, I told the class of the "heart" case prolapse. Of course, I had not mentioned the farmer's name but one of the students blurted out, "that sounds like something my uncle George would do"! A bit of an embarrassing conversation with her....that client was indeed her uncle!

Uterine prolapses are associated with low calcium levels in the bloodstream, prolonged difficult birth, large size of the newborn and sometimes gravity in situations where the mother gives birth with her rear end pointed downhill.

When I was in practice in Abbotsford, B.C., I had a call out to a dairy farm to a first calf heifer that had just calved and prolapsed her uterus. To my horror upon arrival, the heifer was flat on her side, down in the alleyway behind the comfort stalls. The prolapsed uterus was submerged in soupy green feces as the gutter cleaner had not yet cleaned the alleyway. The farmer was quite elderly but after a lot of effort, we managed to get the heifer dragged up into a cleaner comfort stall. Covered in cow feces, I washed the totally "green" uterus to get it as clean as I could before replacement. After getting the uterus replaced, I gave the heifer antibiotics and told the farmer that there was a good chance that she could die from septic infection due to the fecal contamination. I had a call back to his farm about three weeks later; I asked him about the heifer, she was alive and eating but the farmer said to me accusingly "Dr. Schatz, she got infection". (Uterine discharge which could be treated.)

PROLAPSES

One spring (early March) after a warm spell, it rained a lot then turned cold, leaving roads, corrals, etc. very icy. We lived on an acreage just outside of Wainwright and a neighboring couple had built a new home. The immediate community held a housewarming party; it was on a night when my partner Dr. Leitch, was on first call and our associate Dr. Paulsen was on second call. I was on the third call rotation that night, so my wife and I attended the party…..scant chance I would get called out (so I thought).

The rum and coke tasted very good and I admit I was rather "happy". As we left the party (my wife was driving), my unhappy wife snarled at me "how could you drink so much in front of my brothers and sisters-in-law? I hope you get called out, it will serve you right"!

We were only home for about an hour, when my partner phoned; "I've got a Caesarean here at the clinic, Dr. Paulsen is out on a uterine prolapse call south of Chauvin and the Smith brothers at Irma had a uterine prolapse". As I gulped a cup of instant coffee and hurried off to the call, instead of "drive carefully", my wife said to me "serves you right, ha, ha"!

When I arrived at the farm, I was met with an awkward situation; crazy black Angus cow that had chosen to calve by a few bushes half-way down the side of a coulee hill. It was the side of the coulee that did not get much sun so the snow was covered with a slippery layer of ice from the recent rain. Carrying wash water, my doctor's case and I had to navigate down the hillside to where the cow was at…..after three falls (due to the ice of course and not my inebriated state) when I reached the cow, she was not able to stand up. Worse yet, she kept fighting, wanting to make her way facing uphill which put gravity against my efforts to replace the uterine prolapse.

I had put a halter on the cow's head, and with the help of the two farmers managed to get her turned around to face downhill. There is a point in the replacement of a prolapsed uterus, when one has it mostly pushed inside that in spite of the epidural (spinal), the cow will have a stimulus to give a massive strain. It was at this moment, the cow would decide to bellow, throw her head and neck around, send the two farmers flying and struggle around to face uphill again! All of the progress in replacement was lost and the process had to be repeated. This unhappy event occurred about three or four times, I was getting totally exhausted!

There was a cold breeze blowing, I was clad in a rubber obstetrical suit with plastic sleeves and I was getting very cold as well as exhausted. The two farmers were wearing winter parkas as well as mitts....I recall one saying to the other "you know its not that cold out here".

At one point, I had a plastic squeeze bottle with Betadine surgical scrub and when the cow fought her way to a new position, the bottle tipped over on the crusted snow and started to "toboggan" down the coulee hill. "Look at it go", one of the farmers exclaimed!

As the struggle continued to keep the ornery cow in position so I could finally replace the prolapsed uterus, my carry case got tipped over. Some day in the future, some archaeologist may ponder finding Monoject needles, syringes, etc. on that coulee side hill!

After a horrendously long time down in the crusty snow behind the ornery cow, I finally managed to get the prolapsed uterus replaced. Half frozen and totally exhausted, I drove back to our clinic.

In veterinary practice, there were days with few calls and then for some reason, there are days "when all hell breaks loose at once". When I got back to our clinic, Dr. Leitch was doing a Caesarean, Dr. Paulsen was also doing a Caesarean and there was a third obstetrical case awaiting my arrival. One could smell this case all throughout the clinic....the farmer must have missed the cow's early attempts to calve; the breech calf was long dead and

PROLAPSES

well into the process of rotting! Dr. Leitch and Dr. Paulsen were doing Caesareans (fresh calving cases with the delivery of live calves), I had to suffer through delivering the foul stinky rotting calf. At this point my stomach was acting up (perhaps the flu?).... surely not the rum and coke I drank at the party!

I finally had a break to slip home for a shower and a bit of rest. After a bad time at work, a man would expect to be greeted by his wife saying something like "oh you poor dear, have you have breakfast yet"? No way, I was greeted by the words "serves you right, ha ha"!

Over the years, she can forget to pay the telephone bill, pick the twins up from T-ball but she could never seem to forget my night at the party.

It was usually much easier to replace a prolapsed uterus if the cow was capable of standing up for the procedure. However, many of these cases occurred in "down animals" (unable to stand up). Intravenous calcium would enable some of these cases to stand up but many others could not stand up due to a condition known as obturator nerve paralysis. Prolonged pressure of a large calf stuck in the cow's pelvis could bruise the obturator nerves to the hind legs which resulted in failure of the adductor muscles of the hind legs. The cow's legs would splay out to the sides when she attempted to stand up. (Usually, a matter of hours or days and the bruised nerves would "heal" so that standing up was again possible.)

If the farmer had a tractor with a front-end loader handy, ropes could be put on the hind legs of the down cow with the uterine prolapse and the hind quarters of the cow lifted up; this would alleviate pressure of the cow's large rumen stomach and the intestines, making replacement of the prolapsed uterus much easier.

Many times though, when faced with a down cow with a uterine prolapse, if one could get the cow rolled up on her sternum (chest) and pull the hind legs backwards behind her, this would have the effect of elevating the cow's pelvis somewhat, making replacement of the prolapsed uterus easier.

On one occasion when I arrived at a farm, the husband was out seeding his crop and his wife came out with me to a down cow with a uterine prolapse. She was originally from the city but was very keen to learn about cattle and farming. I got the cow in a position with her hind legs out behind her; the young farm wife was very willing to be helpful, so I told her to sit on the cow's back facing towards me and the prolapsed uterus. I told her to hold the cow's tail up as this would "increase the size of the cow's vulvar opening somewhat also making replacement of the prolapsed uterus easier. Busy washing off the uterus and carefully pushing it back in the cow, I suddenly had the feeling that the young wife was "staring daggers" at me. As I glanced up at her, to my immense embarrassment, I noticed that the crotch of her blue jeans had split open! Then I had the thought: oh my God, she thinks I knew that her jeans were ripped, and I deliberately told her to assume that position on the cow. I couldn't finish up that prolapse case soon enough and leave that farm quick enough!

Something I learned the hard way was that one would sometimes deal with a prolapsed uterus case in which the organ was as large as a "tub". This type of case was extremely difficult to lift and manually replace. On one occasion, after struggling for a long time with such a case, I had the idea to make an incision in the uterus....sure enough, a lot of the cow's intestines were inside of the prolapsed uterus. I could reach into the incision, push the intestines back into the cow's body, then suture the incision shut and then replace the much smaller prolapse!

Chapter Eleven

VALUABLE ASSOCIATES

Many valuable associates were part of my practice years at Wainwright.

Dr. Peder Paulsen grew up in Wainwright and worked for Dr. Leitch and I for variable terms. He was primarily interested in large animal work. Dr. Paulsen was very strong physically; I recall him leaning his back into the hindquarters of a 2800- pound Simmental bull and pushing that bull ahead into the headgate! The Wainwright Veterinary Clinic was very fortunate to have the hard -working Dr. Paulsen as an employee.

Dr. Bill Crawford worked for our practice for one year, he would later go on to establish a very successful equine practice in central Alberta. Dr. Gayle Trotter also worked for our practice for about one year. He went on to become a very successful professor at the Colorado State Veterinary College.

Dr. Crawford was noted for one of the most thorough examinations I have ever witnessed, one of his contact lenses dropped out on an old Hereford cow....he spent a very long time looking very closely in the hair of the cow before finally finding the contact lens!

Dr. Trotter played recreational hockey and had the misfortune of breaking a couple of fingers on one hand. The medical doctor decided to use plaster-cast to stabilize the broken fingers. This occurred at the onset of calving season, Dr. Trotter could not do surgeries and many other veterinary tasks. However, he could still place IV catheters so the rest of us veterinarians relegated him to the calf scour ward (akin to a jail sentence in some aspects!)

When Dr. Trotter went to the medical clinic for a check-up, there happened to be some dried fecal stain on his plaster-cast on one finger, a by-product of his working with the scouring calves. There was an Australian nurse who, in spite of a full waiting room of people, she exclaimed "Dr. Trotter have you been picking your nose again"?

In 1980, we hired Dr. Tannis Tupper, a new graduate veterinarian. I recall my first two or three years in practice; I looked like a young kid and it took time to gain acceptance by some members of the public. For Dr. Tupper, there was not only the stigma of looking young but also the fact that she was female.

There was one time when a rancher came in the front of our clinic wanting to speak to a veterinarian; Dr. Tupper was available, but he refused to speak to her, went out and walked around to the back (large animal area) of the clinic to talk to me. Our receptionist called on the intercom to me and I made my way to the front of the clinic. I think we repeated this scenario three times before he relented and would ask Dr. Tupper his questions!

Dr. Tupper was a very proficient small animal veterinarian, but she also took her turn at large animal work. When I left practice to work at Fairview College, she purchased my share of the practice. She provided excellent veterinary service to the Wainwright area until untimely cancer took her life.

VALUABLE ASSOCIATES

Bella Ford served as receptionist and bookkeeper for our practice, and she was the "face of our practice" as she knew many clients. Her gregarious personality was a plus for our practice. When needed we sometimes would ask Bella to assist with a surgery as those were the years when there were no trained veterinary technicians.

There was a time when a client brought in a huge Charolais bull for some corrective hoof trimming. A large animal tilt table was brought into the open alleyway of the large animal area of own clink. The bull (which was restrained in a cattle head gate) was then haltered to the lead/dragged over to the side of the tilt table where he could be restrained with belly bands to the side of the table. Suddenly, the bull went "bullistic" (i.e. on the fight) and broke free, charging at Dr. Leitch and Chuck Hutchinson.

The bull whipped around the large animal counter. At the end of the counter there was a regular sized door with a large diamond shaped window, this door opened to a hallway leading to the front reception area of the clinic. Thinking that he saw an opening, the crazed bull rammed his head through the glass window and in the process, snapped the hinges and lock of the door! He was now in the hallway; at the end of this hallway a similar door with the same type diamond shaped window.

He smashed his head through this window but fortunately the door hinges held fast this time. Poor Bella Ford was sitting at the reception desk when the bull's head smashed through the door window!

Fortunately, the bull turned around and ran back to the large animal area where we were able to lasso him with a lariat rope and get him restrained again. What a close call for Bella! (Luckily glass shards missed her.)

June Fountain cleaned the front area and small animal areas of our clinic, sterilized instruments and also assisted small animal surgeries. I recall one occasion when I was doing a dog Caesarean;

one of the delivered puppies was not breathing and June instinctively gave it mouth to mouth resuscitation! The puppy survived - June was a very dedicated employee.

Anne Woodward also worked as receptionist for many years in our practice. There were times when Dr. Leitch and I were both doing surgeries and our receptionists would have to relay telephone queries to us for Dr. Leitch and I to answer. On one of her first days of work, I recall an extremely embarrassed red-faced Anne coming to the back of the clinic and stammering to me: "there's a guy on the phone who castrated a young bull and now the guts are coming out of the nut bag"! Some farmers were less than delicate in their conversations with our receptionists!

The task of answering phone calls could be very demanding for our receptionist staff, it required sorting out the real urgent calls for us from the calls that were not of an urgent nature. I recall the time when Carmen Granigan started to work at our clinic and she rushed to the back to tell me excitedly "there's a Mr. Spring who has a cow with a Gilbertson stuck on her leg"! (I was able to make the "right" translation.)

Some other valuable employees were Pauline Barber and Gail Ackroyd and large animal assistants Tim Fountain, Bryan Templeton, Chuck Hutchinson, Jim Leitheiser, Bert Kitchen, Grant Ackroyd, Jim Kelly, and George Marcotte. Jim Kelly's first day working as a large animal assistant was an extremely busy day. Poor Jim was very nervous concerning his new job. There were four calving cases arriving at our clinic, one after the other, and we performed four Cesareans on each of these. We had taught Jim to clip the hair off of the surgical areas prior to the Cesarean.

I was talking to a client on the phone while Jim unloaded a Hereford for a farmer. When I got off the phone to examine the animal, Jim in his hurry to please, had the side of the Hereford already clipped. "Jim," I said, "that animal is a steer, we can't do a

VALUABLE ASSOCIATES

Cesarean on him!" (Jim's awkwardness afterwards was only then matched by my awkwardness in explaining to the farmer why his sick steer was clipped for a Cesarean!)

I recall another practice incident involving Jim. One of our associate veterinarians was having an "off" day and he was deriding Jim almost incessantly. The veterinarian was half bent over, making the final skin sutures on a cesarean heifer. Another snide remark was made to Jim. At this point, Jim reached a breaking point; he grabbed a Rochester Pean forceps (it has interlocking teeth on the tips of its jaws) and snapped it shut, locking it on the tissues of the veterinarian's bum! The response was some very very colourful language!

With the eventual evolvement of Animal Health Technology programs at NAIT, Olds College, Lakeland College and Fairview College, Dr. Leitch and I were able to hire two graduate Animal Health Technologists, Marilyn Bell and Brenda Pare. Rather than training local lay people how to assist us, with Marilyn and Brenda, we now had employees with background training who could do treatments for us for our hospitalized animals, assist with surgeries, set up for bull evaluations, etc. The early years for Animal Health Technologists (now denoted as Veterinary Technologists) were fraught with growing pains. There were some veterinarians who worried about the A.H.T.'s taking their work; there were veterinarians who mainly used the A.H.T.'s as cleaning staff. It has been a long, hard and frustrating journey for the veterinary profession to reach today's utilization of veterinary technologists who are now regarded as highly essential for veterinary practices. Again, an amazing positive improvement in veterinary care since I graduated 55 years ago!

Dr. Jim Rattray, Dr. Dick Bibby, Dr. Jim Rhodes and Dr. Dick Weetman worked locums at our practice. Over the years many senior veterinary students worked their senior summer at the Wainwright Veterinary Clinic: Warren Webber, Brian Carpenter,

Maurice Stewart, Rod Niwa, Brian Gordon, Dennis Jackson, JoAnn Schuh, Annette Schmidt-Werner and Janice Anderson. Some other former employees I would like to acknowledge are Elaine Ford, Jennifer Leggett (Killoran), Muriel Steinborn, Shelley Anderson, David, Eddie and Michael Leitch, Terry Pinkowski, Marilyn Booth, Anita Trigg, Debbie McNary, Donna Taylor, Laura Deyell, Faye Oslanski, Faye Krauss, Lana Szoke and Marguerite Rajotte

Chapter Twelve

MUSKOX: A TALE OF WOE

Perhaps a blessing for when I left veterinary practice for the college in the fall of 1987 was the fact that I missed the elk, ostrich, emu and wild boar crazes when Alberta gave the green light to game farming. Our Wainwright practice had about four bison (buffalo) ranchers when I was in practice. One observation was that the bison could be very susceptible to the same internal parasites as affected domestic cattle. I suspect that when the bison were roaming free across north America, that there was little chance of ingesting parasite eggs while grazing as they were constantly moving to new grass. Ranched bison are sometimes kept in confined pastures, sometimes with cattle or the pasture was previously grazed by cattle.

One summer we visited the Head Smashed In Buffalo Jump Museum north of Fort Macleod. Part of the museum's program was a video stimulating how the Indigenous people herded bison over the cliffs…..at one point the video showed a bison with a purple plastic ear tag. Our son Travis was only five years old but he blurted out very loudly "they had ear tags back then"? As an aside, I recognized the tag as belonging to one of our bison clients....he had leased some of his bison to the company that had produced the video.

We had a client who attempted muskox ranching[15]. His idea was that muskox would eat off scrub brush that was taking over pastures and the qiviut (wool) of the muskox could be sold to be weaved into clothing.

Qiviut is the very dense inner wool coat of muskox; this wool coat is protected by a very long hair coat as an outer layer for muskox. The outer layer protects the muskox from wet and snow. In the northern tundra, muskox do not migrate, they are able to withstand very harsh cold winter conditions and survive. When spring arrives, most of the qiviut and long hair coats are shed; regrowth occurs over the summer months. The Inuit people also used muskox for meat.

In the wild, there are classic pictures of muskox forming a protective circle with their heads pointing out when faced with danger. When confronted in captivity in a small corral or pasture, their behavior was to stomp both front feet on the ground, charge forward, stomp the front feet again. This was obvious warning behavior, but the question was always at what point would they stop bluffing and really charge a person!

Our client was able to get permits, hire a helicopter and capture a male muskox calf in the Northwest Territories. The following year he was able to capture and bring back two female muskox calves. That winter the federal government decided that muskox ranching should only be done by the native Inuit people, so he was not allowed to capture any more breeding stock. Thus, he was faced with a slow long process of trying to increase the muskox herd. Also, as the years progressed there was a steep learning curve for both him and I…..there were no lectures on muskox when I was a student at veterinary college!

MUSKOX: A TALE OF WOE

The owner had fenced off some former cattle pasture with chain link fence. He had halter broke the bull muskox calf and it was quite tame when young, however as a mature male in the rut (breeding) season he would charge the chain link fence if someone was on the other side of the fence. The fence would sway in but fortunately it always held!

At one end of the chain link fence pasture, the owner had constructed a wood plank corral, this corral opened to a "V" shaped area to a wood run-way chute; at the end of the chute, he had placed a small cattle squeeze for catching and restraint of a muskox.

Muskox grow very large, thick downward curved horns, as the original animals matured, the owner decided that they should be dehorned. I performed the dehorning procedure similar to one for cattle; restraint in the cattle squeeze, halter and tie the head, local cornual nerve block and local skin block with lidocaine.

The horns were cut off with a wire saw and exposed arteries tied off, pulled or crimped to control bleeding. Then "long acting" penicillin injection to guard off infection and topical wound spray. As compared to cattle, the front of the muskox skull area (horn boss) is very extensive and well developed in muskox. I learned that when dehorning a mature muskox, a very large area of the horn boss must be removed to prevent horn regrowth.

Indeed, one of the muskox cows that I had previously dehorned, had a regrowth of mishapen curved horn that was growing into the side of her face. At this point of time, the veterinary college at Saskatoon had hired a wildlife specialist, Dr. Jeremy Haigh. I had some phone conversations with him, he had expertise on use of a "dart blow gun" and some newer drugs for chemical restraint of exotic animal species. Dr. Haigh had a special permit for a new drug fentanyl (a very powerful narcotic). He had an upcoming trip to Edmonton, and he agreed to stop in

Wainwright and we would to out to the muskox ranch together to dehorn the muskox cow.

The owner had the cow confined in the small plank corral when we arrived. Dr. Haigh shot her with a dose of fentanyl in the blow gun dart; he said "in my experience so far, after a few minutes she will lie down and won't get up until we inject the reversing drug (levalorphan) into her jugular vein"! Sure enough, she laid down and carrying my dehorning supplies, I walked up by her head. Suddenly with a loud snort, she jumped up about one foot from me! This is one time that I was thankful for my homely face as it must have frightened her as she staggered away from me instead of charging! I was just back to work after my knee surgery at this time and the knee was not back to full use as I frantically "hopped" away from her. A few minutes later, she did lay down again and the dehorning/recovery went as planned. While we were working with her, the bull muskox was "bouncing" his head off the nearby wire mesh fence!

One spring the owner called me, one of the muskox calves had an apparent cut on the bridge of its nose. We decided to run the calf into the squeeze, if the cut appeared fresh, perhaps it could be sutured closed. When the muskox calf's head was caught in the bars of the cattle squeeze, the calf jerked its head up and banged the back of its head and neck against the top metal frame. I had just started to examine the cut when the calf collapsed, went down in the squeeze. We quickly released the head as I thought it might be choking itself off. It wasn't acting like a choke case though, it started to kick, stopped breathing. I gave it an injection of epinephrine (adrenaline) but to no avail, it died! When I did a post-mortem, I discovered that although muskox have very protective thick bone structure on the front of their head, the bone at the back of the skull was relatively thin. The muskox calf had fractured (broken) the bone at the base of its skull and fatal hemorrhaging (bleeding) had occurred around the brain stem and first part of the spinal cord, causing pressure and death.

There was another occasion that turned into disaster: a muskox calf with porcupine quills in its muzzle. The calf and its mother were lured into the catch corral, the owner and I were on the outside of the corral waving our arms, trying to get the cow and her calf to run into the chute run-way to the squeeze. The muskox cow was more interested in charging at us, trying to protect her calf. Admittedly both were getting very agitated, suddenly the calf collapsed on the ground. The muskox cow was a danger to us, we couldn't get to the calf. Later the owner had opened up the gate to the rest of the muskox herd and the cow left the calf which was by now.....dead! Post-mortem revealed the cause of death as "capture myopathy"[14], a severe breakdown of the skeletal and heart muscle tissue due to stress. Capture myopathy can occur in a number of exotic animal species; it is the reason why chemical restraint drugs fired by a gun or dart is the safer and preferred way to restrain various wildlife species.

More of a learning curve for raising muskox in captivity; as with bison, in relatively confined pastures they are very prone to developing heavy internal parasite loads. Newborn calves seemed very prone to developing severe cases of coccidiosis! Due to the very long shaggy hair coat of the muskox, bloody diarrhea material would mat on the skin and hair coat around the affected calf's tail and bum. I don't know if the common house fly exists in the tundra up north, but due to the fecal/blood contamination, flies would lay eggs in the affected area. A complicating affliction (myiasis) would occur, that is maggots chewing in the tissues of the affected calves! It became apparent to me that raising muskox in a "farm" situation would require good parasite control, especially for the more susceptible muskox calves.

Sadly, the owner's efforts to establish a muskox herd were severely hampered by the loss of calves. After many years his project was discontinued. I felt somewhat guilty for some of the calf deaths that occurred but again at that time, there was not a body of knowledge about raising them in captivity. Later research at the Western College of Veterinary Medicine greatly improved methods for chemical restraint, nutrition and husbandry of muskox in captivity. Many things were learned the hard way!

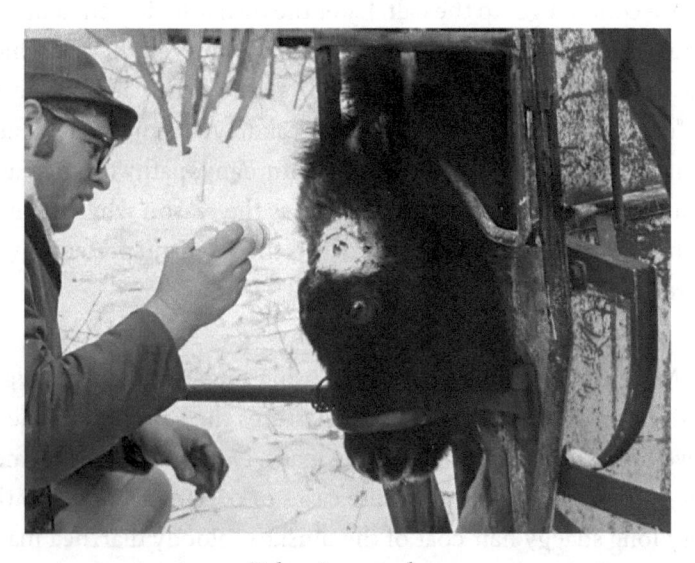

Dehorning a muskox.

MUSKOX: A TALE OF WOE

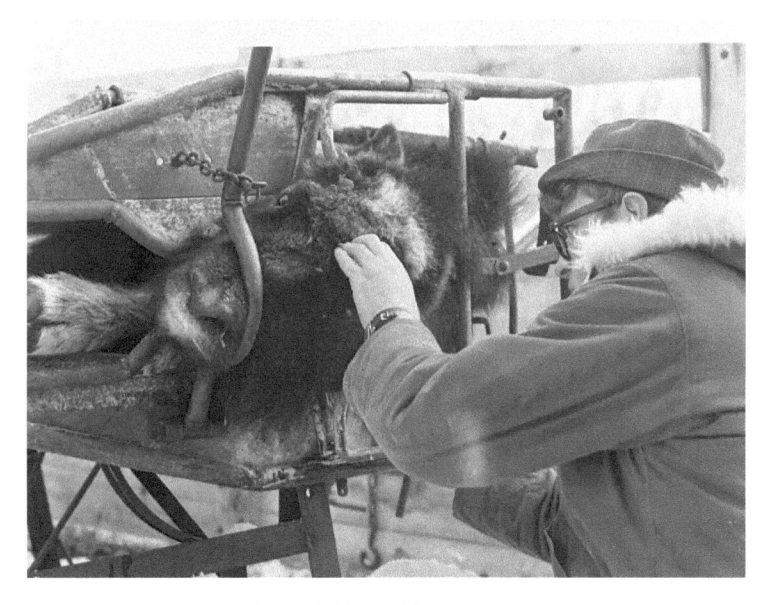

Restraint in a cattle squeeze.

Chapter Thirteen

THE COLLEGE YEARS AT FAIRVIEW

By the time that I had accepted the instructor position at Fairview College in September of 1987, classes were already underway for two weeks. The sensation of suddenly being in charge of classes and labs was somewhat akin to a "cat jumping onto a hot tin roof"! In my naivety, I had many thoughts as to what I had gotten myself into. I was now a "teacher" who had no formal training in educational techniques but I did have the years of practical training in veterinary practice.

The public speaking learned in 4-H was of immense benefit to me in my new instructor role. I developed the habit of telling a practice story or a joke to the class; this perhaps got their attention for a while until my monotone voice lulled then to sleep!

Fellow instructors at that time in the Animal Health Technology Program were Dr. Henry Gauvreau, Dr. Mohammed Ikram, Peggy Johnson, Cynthia Fedoruk and part-time

Fiona Cameron. As well as being instructor, I was appointed Coordinator of the Animal Health Technology Program. Again, little did I know what I had got myself into: budgets, class and lab schedules, student recruitment, etc. Peggy, Cynthia and Fiona were of great help to me in guiding me that fall.

Another startling revelation for me in my new career was the hierarchy of authority and bureaucracy of in essence a government run institution. My predecessor, Dr. Jim Henderson, had resigned from the position of instructor and Coordinator of the Animal Health Technology Program to assume the position of Head of the Regional Diagnostic Pathology Laboratory in Fairview. In retrospect, the college should have appointed either Dr. Ikram or Dr. Gauvreau as Coordinator but it seemed as if the College was worried about backlash if one or the other was named to that role. They both had the benefit of working in the college system which I did not…..I think that there was thus some resentment to me in the Coordinator role. Again, I guess that I was naïve enough to accept that position!

The Animal Health Technology Program was part of the Faculty of Agriculture which at that time included a two-year Agricultural Diploma Program, Beekeeper Technician Program, Farrier Sciences, Equine Studies Program, Ag Mechanics and a Turfgrass Management Program (golf course management). Two very dedicated ladies Marion McDonald and Betty Eddy served as administrative support staff for all of those programs. They would type letters, memos, student instruction guidelines, notes for students, etc.

Marion had a subtle sense of humor and I learned quickly that if she gave an item back for proof reading that one had better do that proof reading meticulously. Case in point, I had a line "students should dress practically for large animal labs"; Marion had typed this instead: "students should dress practically naked for large animal labs". Glad I caught that "Marionism" as my class was all young ladies! Over the years, there were many other examples of Marion's sly humor.

At the time that my employment started, there was a lot of energy and vitality at Fairview College. The College maintained livestock for the Ag programs; commercial beef herd, Purebred Angus herd, Percheron horses, equine program horses, hogs and sheep as well as a dog colony and cat colony. In addition to standard trades programs (general automotive mechanics, heavy duty mechanics, welding, carpentry), there were business programs, adult academic upgrading programs and a transitional vocation program for handicapped.

However, a dark cloud was appearing on the horizon; falling resource revenues and budget deficits meant that the provincial government was mandating cutbacks to college programs as the government sought to eliminate provincial deficits.

Over the following years, this lead to "down-sizing" and the College saw both staff and programs cancelled. Fortunately the AHT program was able to maintain reasonable student numbers and it was not on the "chopping block". There was a time when one college in Alberta put out the proposal that it should be the one and only center of agriculture training in Alberta and the other ag diploma colleges in Alberta should be terminated. Thankfully, I was able to get a number of former veterinary colleagues to write letters of support for the Fairview College AHT program. After a tumultuous period of time, the provincial government dropped that centralized concept for the ag diploma programs in Alberta.

Another revelation that rocked my naivety about employment at a college was the fact that I was an instructor, a member of the Fairview Academic Staff Association (in essence a union). Coming from a background of owning my own business, the mode of thinking of fellow "union" members was certainly something new for me to adjust to.

In spite of all the nuances of organizational chain of authority, internal politics and the like, I decided that my main focus should be the students. The second-year class of AHT students had been taught by Dr. Henderson; not sure what they thought of me as I was certainly a "guinea pig" instructor that fall of 1987. For the first-year class (class of 1989), I think it was easier for them to accept me as an instructor.

There were lectures to give to the AHT students to give them background knowledge in areas such as anatomy, nutrition, husbandry, obstetrics, etc. The second-year class was divided into five groups of four to six students per group; each week each group would rotate through a series of practical labs such as large animal, small animal labs, hematology, microbiology, parasitology lab as well as rotations of work experience at the local private veterinary clinic and the local regional veterinary diagnostic pathology lab. Dr. Gauvreau instructed the small animal (dog and cat) labs while I was responsible for cattle, sleep, pig and horse labs. For illustration one of my labs would be bovine I.V.'s in which I would demonstrate how to take blood from the jugular and tail vein of a cow, how to give injections in those veins; each student would then have a cow upon which to practice those technical skills.

It was a practice of the college to purchase a number of cull cows from various auction markets, these cull cows were kept at the college farm and used for the student labs. The college at that time maintained a herd of fall calving cows so that students could have labs with young calves in the fall session; there was also a late winter/spring calving herd of cows so that young calves were available for labs in the spring session. The flock of ewes at lambing time afforded the students opportunities to work with sheep and often to the great joy of the students, there were cuddly lambs to be bottle fed. Likewise, the hog operation at the college provided young pigs for student labs. John Milne was the farm manager, and he was very helpful and supportive with scheduling and supplying animals for AHT student labs. AHT and agriculture students also had night and weekend calving and lambing checks to gain practical experience.

Arrangements were made to go out to local horse owners with the AHT students for vaccination, blood sampling and deworming horse labs. As well, when the college had an equine studies program, there were those program horses on campus. There was a time when a group of PMU (Pregnant Mare Urine) mare horse farm owners donated weanling foals to the college. These foals provided the equine students with halter breaking, handling, etc. as well there were stud colts that I could use for demonstration horse castration labs with the AHT students.

Public outcry over the humane aspect of the PMU industry as well as advances in synthetizing the hormones required for human medicine lead to the banning and eventual discontinuation of PMU horse farms. In later years at the college, I would arrange for a number of privately-owned colts for the AHT horse castration demo labs.

For a number of years, the college would purchase a number of weaned bull calves with horns. These animals were used for bovine castration and dehorning labs. At one time in the early 1970's, some veterinarians had the idea that castration and dehorning would be tasks for AHT's. In retrospect, this was contentious as the position of the Alberta Veterinary Medical Association was that AHT's were not allowed to diagnose, perform surgery or prescribe treatment. Fortunately, as I mentioned previously, there have been major shifts in the cattle industry towards polled genetics and castration of calves as newborns; it has been a major advance in humane treatment.

Fairview College at that time also maintained a dog colony and litters of puppies would be raised for AHT student labs. Over the years, this practice was discontinued, and program dogs are arranged for from local rescue groups. In the fall of the year, it was also possible to obtain surplus kittens for a cat colony at the college. Each year at the end of the term, some of these dogs and cats would be adopted out to AHT students or the general public.

Across North America, there are many research and pharmaceutical laboratories which utilize mice, rabbits, guinea pigs, hamsters, chickens, etc. for research. Trained personnel are needed to look after these animals thus laboratory animal medicine is a viable career opportunity for AHT's. The college would order in a number of mice, sometimes other lab animal species which were kept for one session at the college for a lab animal course. Most of the female AHT students had to make a great leap of confidence to learn how to handle mice!

Fairview College wrestled with the issue of location in terms of enrolling students, for many years for the AHT program truthfully advertise the availability of animals available on campus. There was always pressure from various sources: "why do you need so many animals, they just stand around all day, what an expense". I tried to tell the naysayers, look "cow #47 needs a week or two rest between being used for blood sampling, Intermuscular injections, etc.". The program animals are at some point sold and there is "recoup" income, as well as the fact that an adequate number of animals provided the opportunity for each student to practice the required skills.

In regards to animal use and perceived abuse, there is an organization, Canadian Council of Animal Care (CCAC) which oversees the use of animals in research and educational institutions. Fairview College was thus subject to CCAC inspection visits and reporting animal usage. A requirement was that the college was to have a functioning animal care committee with at least one public member to approve protocols for animal use for teaching labs, justify numbers used, end use point, etc. For me, a frustration was that from one CCAC inspection panel to another, the membership on the panel varied and sometimes what was OK in a facility last visit was not okay next visit; this made some of my dealings for improvements difficult to present to our college management.

When the Animal Health Technology Program was started at Fairview College in 1974, enrollment in the agriculture programs was in decline. Whatever rooms in the Animal Science building were deemed available were modified for the new AHT program. This worked well at the time. The Animal Science Building was not constructed well; the insulation and heat required upgrades and there was the perennial problem of a flat roofed building: leakage.

For a period of time, I entertained the hope that a brand new AHT building could be constructed on campus; there was a glimmer in time when a private donor may have put up funding to be matched by government grant money. However, in an era of lowered resource revenue, previous government deficits, etc., government grants were being severely slashed. On the other hand, college management was not willing at that time to sanction major renovations to the Animal Science building. It was hard to justify CCAC recommendations for improvements to the large animal area (example, why the expense of stainless-steel countertops and cabinets when the roof leaked on those areas!).

During my first years at Fairview College, the Animal Science Building had one large room (AS 107) which had a tiled floor. There was a raised walkway to rooms AS 111 (small animal), AS 110 (small animal radiology, etc.) and at the south end there was a stairway leading up to a storage room and a viewing gallery for the floor area of AS 107. This viewing area was about five feet wide and had a protective railing for viewers. At the south end of the raised walkway to the small animal area there were countertops and cupboards. There was a walk-in door on the southwest end of AS 107 and on the northwest end of AS 107 was a large doorway through which cows could be chased into the hallway from holding pens (now AS 114, AS 115).

When the AHT program was started, holes for pipes which held removable headgate units were made in the floor of AS 107. This would allow for six cows to be held in headgate units for such labs as bovine epidural (spinals) and mock bovine abdominal surgeries (bovine laparotomies). Local regional nerve blocks for bovine abdominal surgery were also demonstrated and taught here.

The system did work for the purposes stated, however cows produce large quantities of refined grass and water (i.e. manure) and during the course of the lab session, students going to the countertop and cupboards to get syringes of lidocaine would invariably contaminate the walkway to the small animal rooms with cow manure!

In the spring of 1991, before one of the bovine laparotomy labs, one of my AHT students asked me if two of her girlfriends in the business program could watch the lab: "fine" I said, as there was the second floor viewing area. As I mentioned previously, cull cows were purchased from the auction markets and over the years crossbreeding with some of the exotic breeds meant that we started to observe more and more cows that would go "cow crazy" (i.e. go "bullistic" or have a "cowniption") when confined in small quarters.

Just as we finished putting a group of cows in the headgates, one of them started to freak out, and as she threw her head up, she had a stub curled horn which precisely lifted the headgate latch so that she could lurch backwards and out. She was totally on the fight and ready to charge!

Samantha Wilson, AHT, was my assistant for the lab and she managed to quickly get some of the students to safety through one of the doors to the small animal room. I managed to open the sliding door on the northwest corner to allow the rest of the students to run to safety. I thought the crazy cow would run out this door to a hallway that lead to the large animal holding pens. Instead she spotted the stairway up to the second floor and to my amazement she ran up that stairway just like a dog or cat would! At the top of the stairs, she could have turned into the storeroom but instead she turned to make her way towards the viewing gallery, where two terrified girls clasped each other. There was a solid wall at the end of the viewing gallery. I was about to yell at them to jump over the rail to the main floor of AS 107, but somehow, I managed to get part way up the stairway and reach through the guard rail bars with my right hand and slap her on the nose. Luckily, she whipped around and raced back down the stairs to chase me; this time fortunately she headed for the open door to the holding pens.

Although I often told my children and the students that they made my hair turn prematurely grey. It was really that episode with the near miss for injury of the two business students that really turned my hair grey!

At the other end of the Animal Science Building was a large addition AS 144, most of this area was an open sand area but one end had about 14 headgate stalls side by side, where cows could be confined for artificial insemination lab training sessions as well as for a number of AHT labs (e.g. bovine orals, bovine I.V.'s, etc.).

As a result of the near miss with the escaped cow, I was able to get college management to agree to renovations to AS 144: pouring of a cement floor, installation of eight headgate stalls, central gutter, countertops and cupboards and in one corner, a dark room for large animal radiology (i.e. x-ray film development). I was not able to get all that I wanted in the renovations for AS 144 and I didn't get the renovations installed exactly as

I wanted but for many years the system did function fairly well, I think.

Moving the cow labs our of AS 107 meant that most of the area could be converted into a new small animal radiology lab room and dark room for small animal radiology (AS 107A). This freed up FAS 110 for a separate small animal dentistry room (once small animal radiology labs were also held in FAS 110).

At one time, Fairview College offered an abattoir/meat cutting course, but over the course of time, it was discontinued due to the lack of interest. The event of two mega meat packing plants in Alberta meant that these plants trained employees on the job for specific tasks (not the complete slaughter to wrapped product process).

The Animal Science building had holding pens (AS 115) for animals before slaughter, a kill room with scalding tub for hogs, etc.; a meat cutting/wrapping room and a large walk-in cooler. Eventually the large animal holding pens were converted to dog kennels, the kill room was converted into whelping pens for dogs (AS 116) and the meat wrapping room was divided into small animal isolation and three lab animal science rooms (AS 117).

Another area of responsibility as program coordinator was student recruitment. The college had a college Registrar position with the mandate to process student applications for the college's various programs. It was the position of the AHT program that since there was a large number of applications for the available positions in the first year Animal Health Technology class, that the program staff be allowed involvement in the selection process. This had been a source of confrontation between my predecessor Dr. Henderson and the previous Registrar. When I started at Fairview College, a new college Registrar had also started employment, and I inherited the squabble as the new Registrar thought that she should be responsible for all admissions.

However, after discussions with the college President, the AHT program was granted the right to review student applications, decide on accepted candidates, candidates for a wait list and those for outright rejection.

Fairview College was in "competition" for future AHT students with the other AHT colleges in Alberta; NAIT (Northern Alberta Institute of Technology in Edmonton), Lakeland College in Vermilion and Olds College in Olds, Alberta. Many students applied to more than one of these colleges.

We decided to have one or more orientation/tour days on which we would invite prospective students to come to Fairview for a tour of our college AHT facilities, the college and interviews with staff members. Fairview College's northern location was the big disadvantage we faced; the thought was that if the students could see the college, that there was a better chance to "snare" them.

We devised a scoring system to rank students based on high school grades, animal background (i.e. 4-H, animal rescue work, etc.) and the personal interview. The system probably was not perfect, but we tried to follow it to be as fair as we could.

One spring I had made a trip up to the administration building and one of the registration assistants pulled me aside and said "Art, they have drafted a letter of acceptance to a student who is down on the wait list". This was totally a decision of the Registrar and college management. I had not twigged on the student's name but turned out that she was the daughter of a very prominent politician in Alberta. I voiced my objection strongly to management and the letter of acceptance did not go out to that student! We had a system of ranking students on the wait list and it just did not seem fair to make a "jump up" because of politics.

At this point in time, I put in my resignation as Coordinator of the AHT program, I would remain as instructor. In the following months, I did apply for and was offered a position at the Regional Veterinary Diagnostic Pathology Laboratory. However, I declined the offer and decided to stay on as instructor at the college. I had received a somewhat "muffled" letter of apology from College Management and also a "denial" letter from the local MLA. Conversations with the AHT program Coordinator at Lakeland College and Olds College revealed that they had been presented with the same "proposal" for acceptance of that student but their respective college managers stood by their rejection decision without interference. In all of that matter, I think there was a veiled promise of more government funding?

Another feature of our AHT program was to arrange for six-week work practicums for each second year student. Most of the practicums were with private veterinary clinics but we did have students work at places such as the Vancouver Aquarium, Sea World, Calgary Zoo, etc.

For a number of years, NAIT had an arrangement whereby their second year AHT students would come to Fairview College for a six-week "crash" course with large animals. It was often a great challenge to convince a student who had never touched a cow to complete tasks such as passing a stomach tube down a cow's throat! For the most part, the NAIT students did come to enjoy the time at Fairview College. NAIT paid Fairview College for this service but as time went on, NAIT eventually made arrangements for their AHT students to go to farms around Edmonton.

It was also a practice to take the second- year class on a field trip. Two instructors would accompany the students to facilities such as an equine practice, wildlife rehabilitation center, U of A Laboratory, etc. The students would usually decide by class vote what facilities they wanted to tour. It was the year (2007) when I was quite ill with the hairy cell leukemia; the class of that year decided they wanted their tour to be local to Northern Alberta. Arrangements were made to tour a Hutterite colony, buffalo ranch, elk farm and abattoir in Grande Prairie region. With my limited on-line skills, I arranged a motel in Grande Prairie for an overnight stay. That evening, when everyone was booked in the motel, I got a phone call from my daughter and she happened to ask what motel I was staying at. When I told her the name she exclaimed "Jeez dad, what are you doing there? Don't you know that's the prostitute motel"? Oh boy, I had just checked in with a class of 22 female students and a female instructor! (There are a few things I did not tell management about!) So much for selecting a motel just based on rate!

One year the class decided to go to the Western States Veterinary Conference in Las Vegas, Nevada. This was still a time when the provincial government was still putting up matching grant money for fund raisers. With the assistance of Cliff Wagner, Foundation Director of Fairview College at the time, the class held a number of fund-raising events and were able to obtain sufficient funds for registration, hotel and air fare. Dr. Gauvreau, Dr. Ikram and me also attended as chaperones.

In spite of some worries, the students all behaved well and there were no untoward incidents. (One year, previous to my being at Fairview College, Dr. Gauvreau had the chilling experience of a student going AWOL (Absent Without Leave) for the three-day field trip in Edmonton.) Fortunately, she appeared for the bus ride back to Fairview; rumor is her punishment was to clean an area of AS 144 with a toothbrush. Instructors have been known to develop grey hair! (That incident occurred at a time when there was a rape/murder case in south Edmonton.)

A major challenge for the AHT profession for many years was the low wages. Indeed, I had one grandfather ream me out: "why are you promoting such a low paying career? You're misleading the young people who like animals". In recent years, I think veterinary technicians are finally getting better wages and benefit packages when employed in veterinary practices. It has been a long hard road though, many have changed careers or simply dropped out of the profession.

However, there are great success stories such as a number of AHT's who have gone on to veterinary college and became veterinarians. Some started various buisnesses; such as practice management, dog training etc. I am sure that the practical skills learned as an AHT student were of immense benefit when they were veterinary students. Veterinary college teaches one an enormous amount of material, however, I have observed new graduate veterinarians who had a lot of trouble doing a venipuncture. Then again on the other hand, a trained person with excellent technical skills is the whole idea of a veterinary technician.

I ponder back 50 plus years ago to the time when a segment of veterinarians was adamantly against trained animal health technologists/veterinarian technicians to today when there is a high demand for employment for them, especially in small animal practice. While I was a large animal instructor, the position of the Alberta Veterinary Medical Association was very emphatic that the AHT's not be taught bovine rectal palpation and/or pregnancy testing. Fast forward to the 2020's and AHT's with specialized training are now allowed to perform cattle pregnancy testing while under veterinary supervision. The profession has evolved greatly and I'm sure will evolve further in the future.

As the years progressed, sad to say, there were a lot of management decisions on downsizing programs at Fairview College; turfgrass management was given away to Olds College; the beekeeper technician, agriculture diploma, equine studies, farrier science programs plus a number of other programs were discontinued on the basis of low student demand, high costs, etc. There was constant pressure to reduce program costs, then came the move by the provincial government to transfer governance of Fairview College to NAIT in Edmonton. This was supposedly to reduce bureaucracy and increase efficiency. At the start of that five-year experiment, Fairview College reportedly had several million in "surplus savings funds", by the time five-years later that the provincial government gave Grande Prairie Regional College control of the Fairview Campus, the "surplus" funds had disappeared!

After a number of years as a satellite of Grande Prairie Regional College, the Fairview Campus is now a part of Northwestern Polytechnic. I do have to commend G.P.R.C. management; the "bullet was bit" and extensive repairs to the roof of the Animal Science building were made, the building was re-insulated as well as new heating/ventilation systems. A complete renovation of AS 144 was completed with new cattle handling equipment, an equine anesthesia recovery room was constructed in AS 144 as well as new stainless-steel counter tops and cupboards. Likewise, improvements were made to the small animal examination/treatment room, surgery suite, etc. to finally come up to CCAC standards. GPRC in my mind made a commitment to a long-term future of the AHT program at Fairview Campus.

In the summer of 1995, I was able to have Fairview College sponsor the RCMP Musical Ride. The event drew a crowd of about 3000 people and a few thousand dollars of income was thus dedicated to an Animal Health Technology Scholarship Fund for student assistance.

There was a time when Fairview College would host an annual awards night for students and the donors of various awards. This event was well attended and provided an excellent connection to people in the Fairview area.....unfortunately it was discontinued due to perceived cost issues.

It was sometimes said that "the Animal Health Technology Program (mostly female students) and the Turfgrass Management Program (mostly male students) were complementary programs"! Indeed over the years students from these two programs did find their soulmates! Of note is also the fact that some AHT graduates married local Fairview men and have raised their families in the Fairview area.

One of the courses I taught to the AHT students was Obstetrics and Reproduction of domestic animals. At the start, it was a bit of a hurdle for me to get over teaching this topic to a class of young ladies. I tried to be just straight forward and factual without saying anything really sexist.

However, there were sometimes occasions where some of their comments left me a bit embarrassed. At one time during a bovine orals lab, I was having the students practice giving boluses (large pills) to cows. The group of cows at that time were rather wild and not above throwing their heads at a person. I had instructed the students how to quickly step in beside a cow's head, get the side of their body right against the side of the cow's head and reach over the cow's face with an arm to get control of the cow's head. In spite of this one cow swung her head and the top of the cow's head hit the front of the student's chest. In pain, she stepped away from the cow and while rubbing her chest, she yelled "expletive expletive! Dr. Schatz". "By the time we are done with these son of a bitchin cows, we won't have any expletive boobs left"! What could I say?

On one occasion, during a sheep lab with the AHT students, we were using young lambs, one student would restrain a lamb in front of her chest and between her legs. A classmate then would do the procedure of getting a blood sample from the jugular vein of the lamb. One time a particular lamb starting to whip it's tail around back and forth right at the level of the crotch of the girl holding the lamb. She shrieked "Jeez, better than a man"! What could I say?

During the years when the AHT students went on rotations at the local private veterinary clinic, Dr. McWatt related the story of the time that he was out on a farm call with an AHT student. Dr. McWatt was examining a pen of young pigs; one of the pigs had a scrotal hernia (loop of intestine inside the scrotal sac beside the testicle). He told the student to palpate the hernia and said to her "did you ever feel anything like that"? "Yes", she replied, "last Saturday night"!

Overall those stories contrast with the fact that for some of the AHT students, topics of reproduction would cause them to blush.

Almost every year the AHT, agriculture, equine and turfgrass students would host a fund- raising event in the Hawker Pavilion. A dunk tank was a yearly feature of that event and I volunteered for dunk tank duty each year. For some reason, all the students wanted a turn at hitting the target and dumping me into the tank! I usually had a 60 cc plastic syringe and would squirt water at them to really put them into a "get even" mood!

Over all the years I instructed at the college, I had a constant worry about any of the students getting severely injured during the large animal lab sessions. I'm sure most of the students who were small animal orientated hated me at times for insisting that they practice a number of procedures on rather mean wacko cows. As I mentioned previously, cows were purchased by an order buyer at auction markets, in spite of instructions to buy quiet cattle we did end up with some bad acting cows; as much as possible I tried to avoid using them or I would try to use the crazy ones myself as demonstration cows. Although a number of students over the years did sustain kicks and various bruises, I never had a student experience a broken arm, broken ribs or broken leg.

Each year at the end of the session, I always felt a great relief that it had passed without a serious injury to a student.

A somewhat startling revelation: it was Easter of 1988, during my first year as instructor at Fairview College. One of the twins said to Eileen, "Mom, why is Dad home today"? This pointed out that in all of my years in veterinary practice, Easter always occurred during calving season and usually during the busiest part of the calving season. It dawned on me that due to the nature of my work, I had "missed Easter" with my kids when they were at the youngest ages of their lives.

I do not fully recall the circumstances but somehow, I acquired the nickname Dr. Danger Schatz while working as a college instructor. One of the farm crew once teased me by referring to me as Dr. Death Schatz. One of the students thought that he had said Dr. Danger Schatz. Another slant to this story is that once I was in a pen dealing with a group of crazy cattle and the students thought that I was in danger, hence the nickname Dr. Danger Schatz. Regardless of its origins, that handle seemed to pass on from year to year to successive classes of students.

Much as I worried about students getting injured in the animal labs, I also worried about them when they travelled to and from Fairview College; some of them had to drive very long distances and the return trip after the Christmas break which often occurred in severe winter weather with icy roads. Two students from one of our sister Alberta AHT colleges were killed in a vehicle accident when going back to college.

A very tragic accident occurred for one of Fairview College's AHT graduates. She was struck by lightning while out on a baseball field. In spite of being revived twice she succumbed to her injuries. I remember her as a good student and a nice person.

In addition to fellow AHT staff I have already mentioned. I would like to express my gratitude to a number of other AHT instructors, Lab Technicians and Lab Assistants on staff for bearing with me and their dedication to the program while I was employed at the college. My apologies if I have missed a number of people, however, kudos to Dr. Susan Klassen, Dr. Ron Smith, Dr. Marliss Anderson, Dr. Ursula Jedra, Dr. Rick Vanderkove, Dr. Terill Udenberg, Rhonda Shaw, Karlee Worobetz, Trish Hulobowich, Anne McIntyre, Bev Milne, Wanda Massicotte, Bev Wieben, Susan St. Croix, Karen Lesnick, Tanya Sooley, and Nichole Boutilier. Lois Saville, Nadia Nichol and Lin Roy provided excellent administrative support for the AHT students and staff after Marion and Betty retired.

I retired from the college June 30, 2010.... from what I had first envisioned as one year at the college had become a stay of 23 years. Although I enjoyed the interaction with the students, I felt that the time had come for a change. Among the 600 or so AHT, agriculture and equine students I had taught over the years, there have been a number who stop in for a visit if they are ever passing through Fairview. A few send a Christmas card and a fair number keep in touch with me through Facebook. It is nice to hear about their careers, families, travels and achievements.

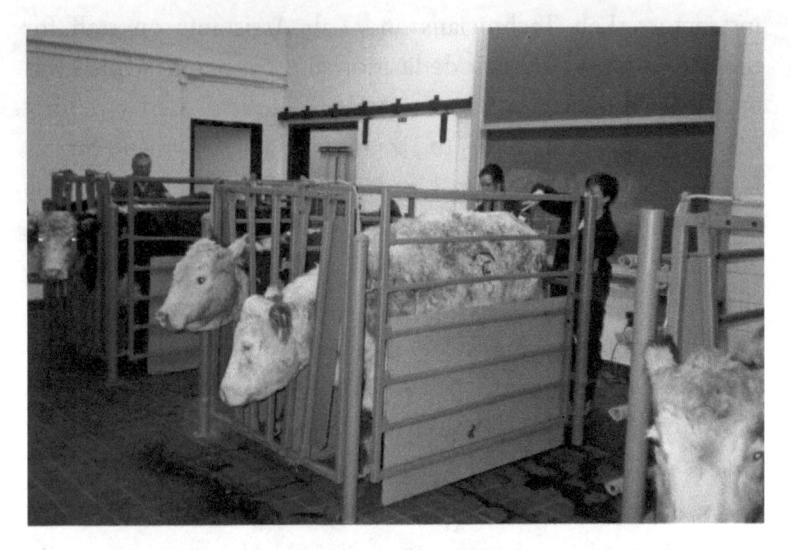

Epidural lab session in AS 107. Renovations in later years had the head stalls moved to AS 144 and the room AS 107 was converted to small Animal Radiology room

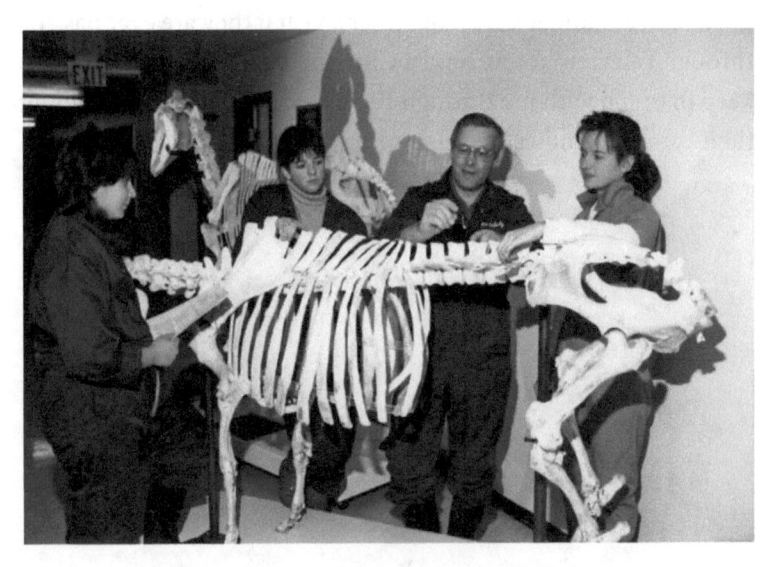

Using cow skeleton to demonstrate boney landmarks for paravertebral nerve blocks

THE COLLEGE YEARS AT FAIRVIEW

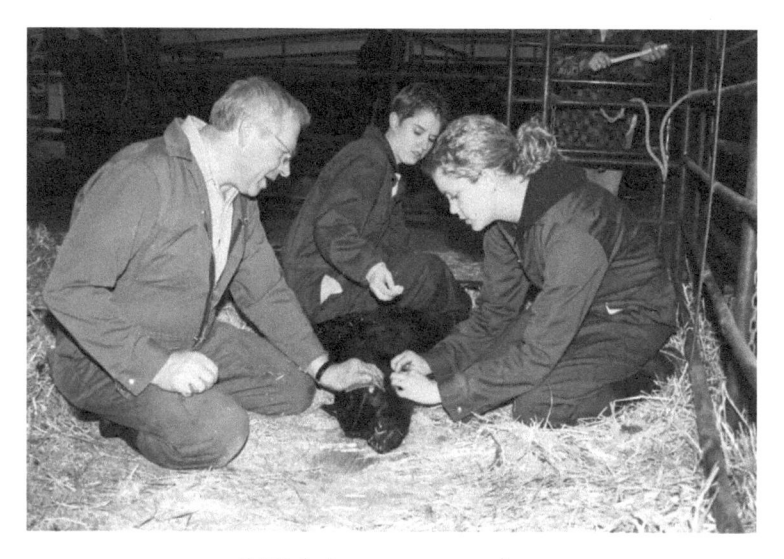

Calf Lab: Intravenous procedures

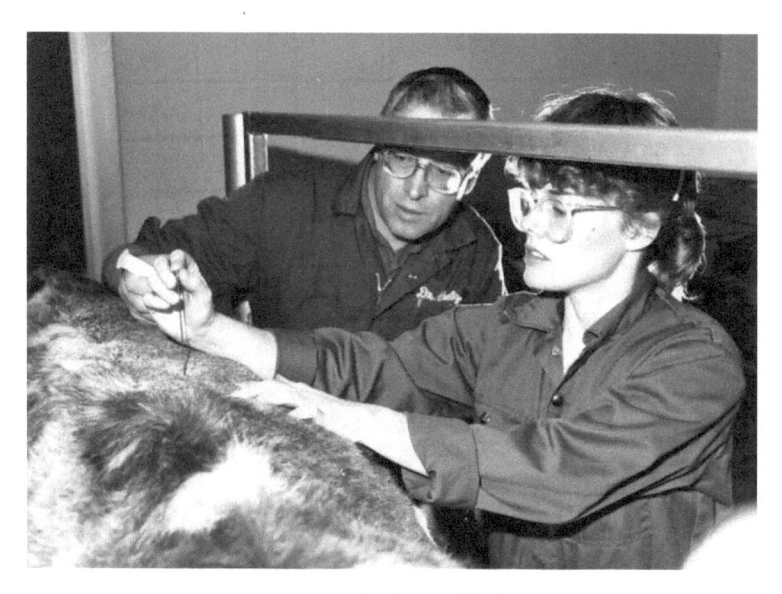

Paravertebral nerve block

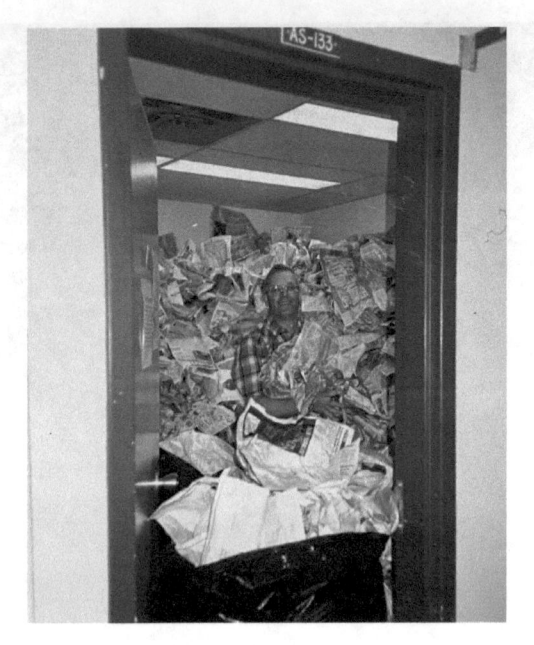

One class decided that I needed lots of newspapers to read!

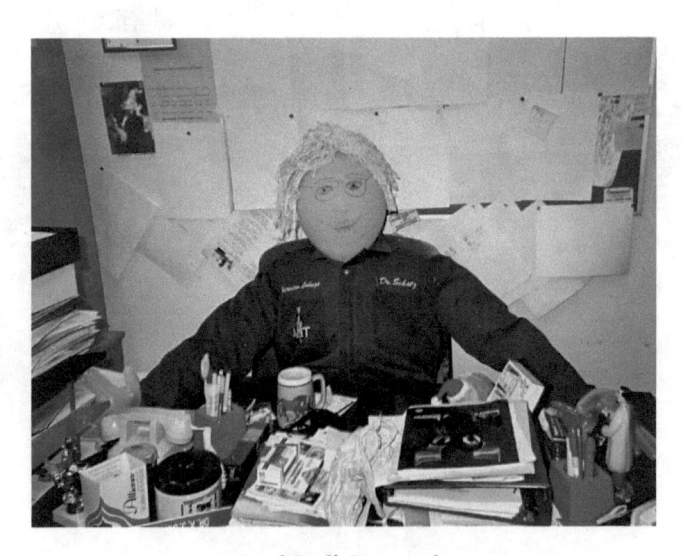

April Fool's Day prank:
The students rearranged "me" and my office

THE COLLEGE YEARS AT FAIRVIEW

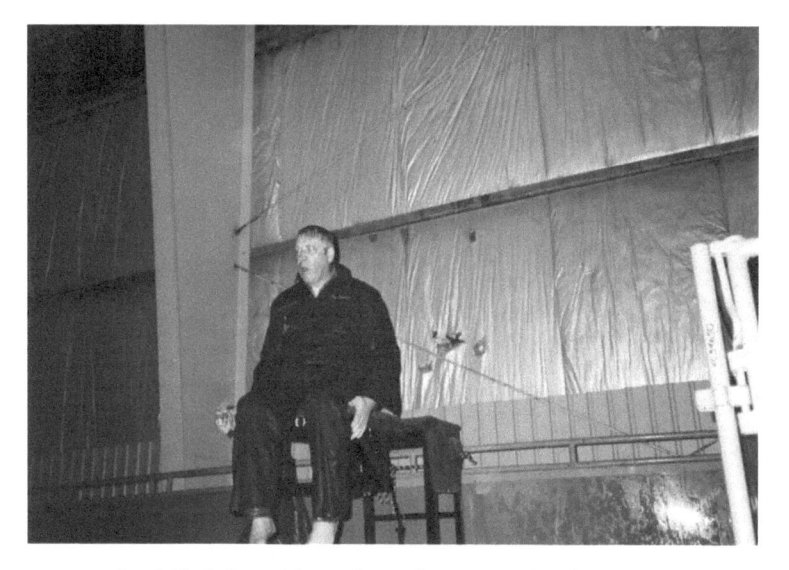

Dunk Tank Duty: The students always wanted to drown me!

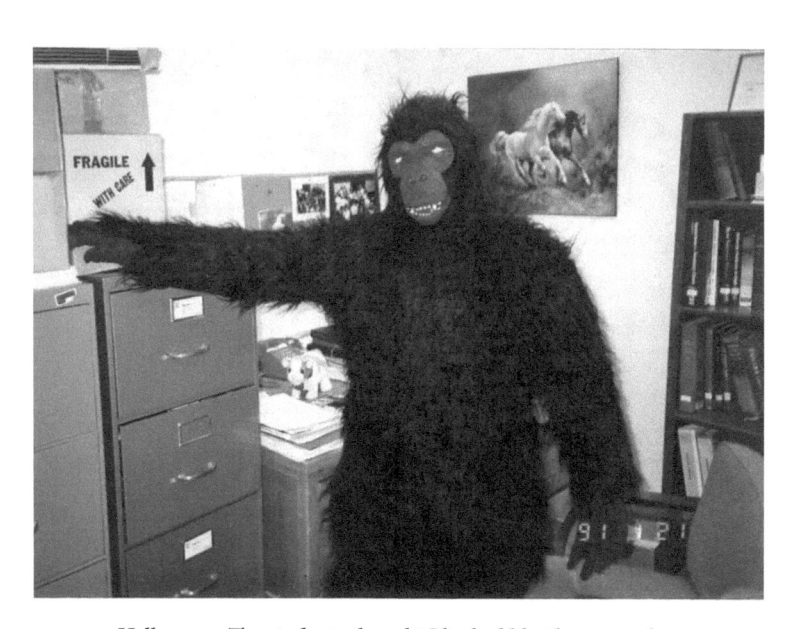

Halloween: The students thought I looked like this every day.

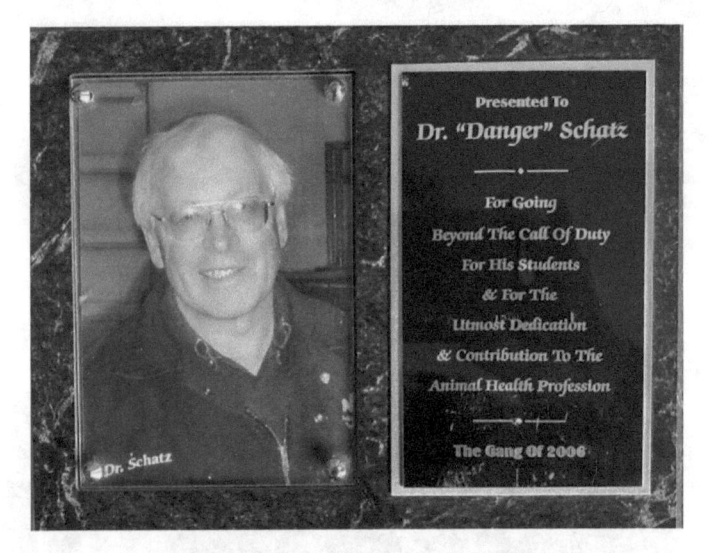

Plaque presented by the class of 2006

THE COLLEGE YEARS AT FAIRVIEW

True celebrities are a rarity. I am not talking about the modern variety that is in the news and magazines bombarding us with useless bits of information. I am talking about People that personify an idea or an institute. People we may hear about long before we may ever meet them, who can change lives and who we take along for our journey, forever linked to that period when we met. The person I am introducing today is to me a true celebrity. I personally first heard about his exploits in 1989, when brand new to Canada I was told tales about this man, who had left the Wainwright area 18 months before, to venture out to educate AHT at a college way up North.

At Fairview Dr. Schatz influenced over 23 years of Animal health students, equine students, ag students. And an overwhelming majority of them would agree with me that Dr. Art "Danger" Schatz is an icon, his name and face linked to the Fairview AHT program in such a bond that it is somewhat hard to believe that it would not continue forever.

How do you describe what Dr. Schatz did for this college, its students and its staff, without cutting into his retirement time by going on and on? I know I cannot compete with his legendary jokes, so I settled on two words: He Cares. Dr. Schatz cares about the college, he cares about the program, he cares about the people here, he cares about the animals, and most of all he cares about the students. And for that we cannot thank him enough. Can I have a big applause for Dr. Art Schatz

Student Centred
- Accountability
- Integrity
- Innovation
- Respect
- Passion

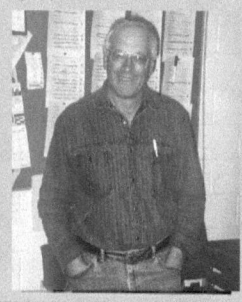

Retirement announcement 2010

Chapter Fourteen

MORE PRACTICE REFLECTIONS

One area of cattle practice is to perform what we call breeding soundness evaluations on bulls before the breeding season. A high calving rate is one of the most important goals of a successful beef cattle operation. As veterinarians we assess the overall physical health condition of a bull, examine and palpate the reproductive organs for abnormalities, followed by collection of a semen sample for microscopic examination. Motility (movement) of the sperm cells and then morphology (shape or appearance) of individual sperm cells is assessed using a microscope.

The most common way to obtain a semen sample from a bull involves the use of a device called an electroejaculator: a rectal probe with three long vertical electrodes is placed inside the bull's rectum. The probe is connected by an electric cord to a control box. Electrical stimulations of variable time and intensity causes impulses through the wall of the bull's rectum to the underlying accessory sex glands (prostate seminal vesicles) as well as the "pelvic portion" of the bull's penis. If all goes well with the process, there is stimulation, protrusion and ejaculation so that a semen sample may be obtained for evaluation.

One day a young couple brought in a very fat yearling Hereford that they had just bought for a breeding soundness evaluation. There were about four other clients waiting for me by the chute area. The bull was not responding well to the electroejaculation stimulation (no protrusion of penis, no ejaculation). At this point the young wife said to her husband "Jeez Sam, he's no better than you"! The other clients broke into prolonged laughter while the husband glared at her and the air seemed to turn frosty! (Not sure if she said that as a joke or if she meant it?)

As a side note, the use of the electroejaculator has been severely criticized by animal welfare advocates as being inhumane. Certainly in my early years of practice, the old style ejaculators did cause some bulls to bellow, struggle and even lie down. The newer ejaculators in use in practice today have improved technology and adverse signs of pain to the bull are now seldom observed.

Once we had a client who was raising Chianina cattle (a very large, tall cattle breed native to Italy). He had an extremely big Chianina bull and had experienced a poor calf crop from this bull. The bull was too big, tall and ornery to load and bring to the clinic, so he asked me to come out to his farm to do the bull evaluation there. At the farm, the bull was too big to fit into the farmer's squeeze chute, but the farmer had him blocked off in a tall wood plank alleyway with a big fence post behind the bull to keep it confined.

There was a company that had just manufactured a supposedly new superior bull ejaculator, the "Electrojac"; it would produce, starting from low intensity, a series of automatic stimulations to the probe in the rectum (older ejaculators had hand knob

MORE PRACTICE REFLECTIONS

manual controls). All of the electronic circuitry was inside of the Electrojac probe with a cord leading to an on-off switch.

We had just purchased the Electrojac for our practice and this was my first occasion to use it. I had completed my overall examination of the bull (he was almost six foot tall at the withers and I'm sure over 3000 pounds weight). I placed the Electrojac probe in the bull's rectum, then turned on the power. The bull gave a massive bellow, reared up on his hindlegs and threw his front legs over the top of the wood chute. His weight broke the wood planks, and he galloped off out into an adjoining bush pasture! On the cord to the probe, there was something called a "break away adapter"......it disconnected when the bull jumped out, leaving the expensive probe in the bull's rectum as the bull took off running.

With the owner, I spent most of the rest of the afternoon walking the pasture to find where the bull had finally pooped the probe out onto the ground! Veterinary practice does cause early growth of grey hair for veterinarians!

Over the following years, improvements were made to the Electrojac as newer models came to market. Never did get the evaluation of that bull completed as the owner opted for a slaughter on the farm for meat for that bull! In Italy I think the farmers put in nose rings in the Chianina cattle at a very young age and halter broke them as calves so that the cattle are manageable. In my experience, raised under our Western Canadian range conditions, Chianina cattle were very flighty and unmanageable.

As an aside, in the early years of the exotic cattle boom, a group of investors had imported nine yearling Chianina bulls to Canada. They were called the "F" bulls as their registered names all began with the letter "F". By use of artificial insemination, half-blood female Chianina females were produced by breeding to our domestic Herefords, Angus, etc. Then the half-blood

Chianina heifers were A.I. bred to one or another of the "F" bulls (i.e. not their father "F" bull). To the dismay of farmers, some of the three-quarter blood Chianina calves that resulted were born with umbilical fissures! In this condition, the skin and muscles of the ventral midline do not grow together, leaving the calves born with their intestines and stomach out in the open. Instead of being worth thousands of dollars, their calves had to be euthanized (or they died at birth). Further investigation revealed that the imported "F" Chianina bulls were related to each other, and they were carriers of recessive genes which could cause the deformed calves. Ironically, one of the investor group was a geneticist at the U. of A.; again I think the Italian farmers knew what they were getting rid of!

I recall a client who had purchased two very expensive Charolais breeding bulls in January. Near the end of March of that year he called me out to his farm to perform breeding soundness evaluation of those bulls.

Upon physical examination of the first bull I was perplexed as the bull's testicles were somewhat swollen, "hot" and painful upon palpation. More bewildering, there were scabs on the skin of the scrotum with small hard lumps below the scabs. The bull's testicles would not move up and down in the scrotum. (For optimal sperm cell production, the testicles need to be "down" from the body to be somewhat cooler than body temperature.)

When I examined the second bull, the findings were similar to those of the first bull. Very peculiar! Curious, I picked off the crust of the scab and upon a bit of pressure being applied I squeezed out an AIR RIFLE PELLET!

Turns out that the bull's owner had given his young son an air rifle gun for Christmas. "Junior" admitted to numerous occasions when he snuck up behind the bulls at the feeder and shot the bulls in the "nuts"! He evidently thought it was very humerous to watch the bulls bellow and jump when the pellets hit!

MORE PRACTICE REFLECTIONS

Inflammation and scar tissue reaction to the pellets caused the scrotal skin to adhere to the testicles. Needless to say, the father was not amused with his son's performance as two bulls worth thousands of dollars were ruined for breeding purposes! The bulls were sold for salvage slaughter at a much reduced value.

The unpleasant task of having to euthanize an animal can be a drain upon a veterinarian's mind. Many times, we face the sad situation when the owner requests euthanasia of a pet because real or perceived behavior issues of the pet. Those cases are very hard for a veterinarian, we sometimes tried to find someone to adopt the pet but often we followed the owner's request, with the thinking that it was better than some other options that the owner may undertake on his/her own volition (such as shooting, drowning, abandonment, etc.).

Of course, many euthanasia requests were for severe injuries, cancer, age related problems, etc. Once I had a client bring in his saddle horse. It had a very severe limp and a swollen left stifle joint. Examination and x-ray films revealed the patella bone (equivalent to human kneecap) was shattered into multiple pieces. Any repair would involve wiring or pinning or screwing the bone fragments together and because of movement and rather poor blood supply to the patella. The chance of such extensive surgery being successful was very low. The most humane course was euthanasia. The owner was very distraught. He said he would take his horse back home and think it over.

About midnight, I received a phone call from his wife "Art", she said, "Pete's been drinking and had decided to have Rocky put down. I'm sorry about the hour, but he wants it done tonight. He is in an awful state of mind".

As I was going out to the farm, a thunder and lightning storm started to roll in. The owner had a backhoe and had dug a trench for burial of the horse. There were cracks of lightening in rapid succession by this time and lots of thunder. I required someone to hold the horse steady while I injected a lethal dose of concentrated barbiturate in the horse's jugular vein. There was just the owner and I and he refused to hold the horse for me as he was crying, swearing and obviously under the influence as he was downing a "26" of whiskey straight!

If an animal moves or struggles when one is giving an injection of barbiturate, and the needle comes out of the vein and if a small dose of barbiturate has been injected that can induce a panic state in the animal. The thunderstorm was getting worse, and torrents of rain were coming down.

The trench the owner had dug sloped down to a deep end. I thought I'll lead Rocky down to the deep end and if I had a problem, that he would at least be somewhat confined by the trench. Rocky was a great horse, and I led him down into the trench with no issue. I had driven my car so that the headlights shone down the open end of the trench so that I would have some light. The injection went smoothly and Rocky went down. I waited for some time so that I could ensure that Rocky was dead and remove his halter.

Suddenly I heard the tractor backhoe engine running; the backhoe bucket was swinging over the trench and lumps of dirt were falling down by the dead horse and myself! The swinging of the bucket was very erratic! Most of the swinging was coming from the more shallow end of the trench. I started to yell at the owner in the backhoe, but the rain and thunder probably drowned out my yells.

My older brothers worked in construction and one of them related the gruesome story of a worker who had his head split open by the backhoe bucket! I attempted to climb out of the deep end of the trench, but the sides of the trench were too slippery because of the rain. Visions of being buried alive with a dead horse flashed through my frantic mind! The backhoe bucket swung away from the top of the trench at one point, and I desperately hopped over Rocky's body and made a frantic run out of the shallow end of the trench!

I banged on the door of the backhoe cab and gave the inebriated owner a bit of my mind. "I thought you were back in your car", he blurted.

There is a related ironic bit of karma to my story. One of my friends in Wainwright worked part-time for the local funeral home. He had the experience of being asked (just before the end of the funeral service) to go out to the cemetery and check the gravesite. There had been a heavy rainstorm the night before and while Garry was checking the grave a portion of its wall and Garry fell into the open grave. Dressed in a suit and mindful of keeping a good appearance, he discovered that the muddy grave walls were slippery! He struggled to get out and had visions of the funeral party coming out to find him trapped in the grave! (He did manage finally to get out.)

I laughed and laughed when he told me that story.... about two weeks later I had a similar experience with a dead horse in a trench! Karma knows no limits!

Along the lines of euthanasia, there was a time when a liner carrying a load of purebred Polled Herefords had a bad accident. Several of the animals were killed outright. The attending RCMP officers had elected to shoot several badly injured animals. When I arrived, I determined that there were a number of animals that were O.K. other than one yearling heifer. She was up and standing but had a large open wound on the left side of her chest. Arrangements were made with a local farmer to haul her to our clinic where I hospitalized her for treatment. She had obvious broken ribs; I debated if I could wire them together or if confined stall rest would aid healing. There could have been some internal organ damage or perhaps her response to pain, for she would not eat. Daily treatment involved passing a stomach tube to pump in water, propylene glycol, molasses for maintenance nourishment. After three weeks she was still not eating; I had a telephone conversation with the owner. "Alright", he said, "if she's not eating by tomorrow morning, go ahead and euthanize her". Next morning when I went into the clinic, to my amazement, she was eating! A few days later, I sent her home.

As mentioned previously despite having a clinic it was still necessary to make some farm calls. GPS and Google maps were in the future so as veterinarians we relied on verbal directions or municipal maps for guidance to drive to farms. Alas, the verbal directions or even there maps were not always infallible!

One July day a farmer called that he had a sick Holstein steer. He had a job off the farm as he requested a farm call; he gave me directions as the which municipal road to turn off from Highway 14. "So north on the gravel road" he said, "you'll see a slough and the road curves around the slough, my farm is the first one on the right after the curve. The steer is in the barn."

Directions seemed straight forward and at the farm I found a Holstein steer in the barn. Although the steer had a bit of a nasal discharge, he ran and bucked around his pen and playfully tried to head bunt me. I put a halter on him and upon physical examination of him I thought "gee, he's perfectly normal, maybe the owner is just paranoid." I gave the animal a fresh flake of hay and he readily started to eat it.

After supper that night (when the owner was home from work" I gave him a phone call that his steer was perfectly healthy. The owner snarled "NO, he's not… he's grunting, breathing heavily and not eating!"

After I gasped and sputtered for a while some further questioning of the owner revealed that further north on the road was a very large slough and long curve in the road just before his farm.

MORE PRACTICE REFLECTIONS

He didn't consider the previous small slough and small curve to be significant!

I made a hasty evening call out to the "correct farm" and the barn was the "correct Holstein steer." (At my own time and expense.)

Talk about crazy circumstances and coincidences (two sloughs, two curves, two Holstein steers in the barn).

A lesson was learned; one must always be careful of directions given according to physical landmarks!

One day a tall, tanned "Marlboro" type cowboy from the Czar area brought in a litter of Blue Heeler puppies for vaccinations. When I vaccinated one of the puppies, it started to whimper. The rancher reached over, picked up the puppy in his arms and started to baby talk to it "aw did he stick that gweat bwig needle in you?" he said. My assistant lost it and gave out an audible giggle…I have to confess, I nearly lost it myself!

I recall another bite my tongue experience; I was talking to a couple, the wife had a young female poodle. At this point, she did not want to have her dog spayed (ovariohysterectomy) as she thought that in future she might want to let the dog have puppies. They had a couple of male cattle dogs and on the other hand she was worried about her poodle getting bred to one of them. I went through the onset and duration times and signs of estrus for a female dog, explaining that she would have to maintain about a three week lock down of her poodle. At that era of time, a company was promoting a product which if given to a female dog for a number of days would eliminate the estrus odor in her urine and thus eliminate attracting male dogs. I had just finished explaining this option to them, when the husband turned to his wife and said "that's what you need"! (I think his remark was in context to the dog?)

We had clients who had a female donkey. I received a call to look the donkey. When I examined her, she was very lame on the hind legs. Closer examination revealed broken off porcupine quills in the pastern/fetlock areas of her hind legs. I gave the donkey an anesthetic and spent a considerable amount of time probing for broken off quills. An antibiotic injection and tetanus antitoxin was given to prevent infection. Over a week later, the owner's wife called, as the donkey was limping again. On that visit, I was able to locate and remove a few more quills and fervently hoped that the donkey had learned not to kick a porcupine again.

Back in town, it was noon and I decided to stop at the post office and check for mail. The area around the post office on main street was quite busy with a number of people. From across the street, the owner (husband) of the donkey spotted me and yelled out, "Schatz you bugger, I heard that you were out looking at my wife's ass again"!

A client of ours had a Dachshund dog, Fritz, that was vomiting, lethargic, dehydrated and had pain when the abdomen was palpated. A round hard mass was palpated. Upon abdominal surgery, I removed a marble that was stuck in Fritz's small intestine. Fritz made an uneventful recovery. The owners asked for the marble back for "show and tell" with their friends. About three weeks later, the owners brought Fritz back….. and yes, he had swallowed the marble again!

Another awkward reflection was the time when I went out to a 5:00 a.m. uterine prolapse call. When I finished replacement and treatment of the uterine prolapse, the farmer said to me "come in for coffee and breakfast, I told my wife to make those when you arrived". As I was rather tired from a previous night call, I agreed to his offer.

Upon entering the house, I was soon filled with vast regret. His wife had evidently fallen back to sleep; coffee and breakfast were not ready! The farmer started yelling at his wife as she started coffee and breakfast….. about every minute he would yell at her "you got coffee ready yet"? There was an atmosphere of ice in the air in that kitchen….. I wished I wasn't there as the two exchanged frosty words. After the umpteenth time that he yelled at her about the coffee being ready yet, she grabbed the coffee pot and in-a-flash poured hot coffee on his head! He jumped up, and bellowed "expletive, expletive, woman, be reasonable"!

She had a big smirk on her face as he continued to curse and rub his head. I think I felt as uncomfortable as him.

When I was in the practice in the Fraser Valley at Abbotsford, the general tone was to finish your work on the farm call and leave. I was utterly astounded by the fact that in the Wainwright, Edgerton, Chauvin, Irma, Czar, Hughenden, Amisk, Hardisty, Metiskow, Cadogan, Provost areas when out on farm calls there was almost always an offer to come in for coffee or a meal! To this day, I am still grateful for the hospitality of the clients in the Wainwright practice area.

During calving season, when we were doing night call cases in our clinic, members of the local RCMP (Royal Canadian Mounted Police) detachment would often make stops at our clinic to observe Cesareans, calvings, etc. as a bit of a break from their night patrols. We always had coffee on at our clinic so that was always available to the RCMP. Needless to say, we got to a first name basis with the RCMP members.

One day I was on my way back from calls in the Chauvin area; yes I was speeding as I was over two hours late on a booking for bull evaluations at Hughenden. With my mind preoccupied with being late, I came upon a line of four vehicles ahead of me. There was a long clear stretch of highway 14 ahead of me so I tramped on the gas to pass all four vehicles; as I was whizzing by them, I glanced to my right and was jolted by the fact that the third vehicle was an RCMP cruiser! "Oh my God", I exclaimed to myself, "I just passed a cop"!

The RCMP officer flashed on the cruiser's lights and siren and pulled me over. "Art", he yelled, "what the hell were you thinking"? Embarrassed, I mumbled my excuse about being late for another call. We had treated his wife's dog at our clinic so he knew me from that aspect as well as from the night stops at our clinic. He gave me a warning lecture but didn't give me a speeding ticket. Whew, dodged a bullet on that one!

A sad reality of our North American societies is the perpetual problem of stray dogs and cats. In spite of various animal control by-laws, licensing, animal shelters and spay and neuter programs, various towns and cities struggle with the issue of strays from time to time. Millions of unwanted dogs and cats are euthanized each year in North America. It is a frustrating problem.

Sometimes there are people who take "matters into their own hands", indeed, in Wainwright there were occurrences of someone poisoning dogs. The usual poison was strychnine, a poison widely used in farm areas for the control of the Richardson ground squirrel (gopher). This poison could be used to lace a portion of hamburger meat or a hot dog wiener and put out around town to poison dogs. Often the problem dog was not a victim, and the practice was also a potential danger to a small child.

Strychnine acts by over stimulation of nerve impulses to muscles of the body: the affected animal goes into spasms of muscle contractions with death occurring when the muscles of respiration "lock" in contraction. In our practice, we sometimes had to perform post-mortems of dogs that died suddenly. Lab test results would be positive for strychnine poisonings. We also had cases of live dogs in spasmodic convulsions as clinical cases; we were able to save the lives of some of these by stomach lavage and/or controlling the spasms by intra-venous barbiturate drugs.

The problem of poisoned dogs seemed to vary from time to time of year. No perpetrator was ever caught in-spite of efforts by local townspeople and the RCMP.

For a time, the Wainwright Veterinary Clinic served as animal pound for the town of Wainwright. There was a point in time where the town council decided on a policy to pay $10.00 for each stray dog or cat brought into the pound. A couple of the local drunkards seized upon this golden opportunity for funding their drinking problem. The issue came to a "firey head" when a local lady put her old blind Pekinese dog out on her front lawn. She went back into her house and happened to look out her front window to see one of the local drunkards snatch her dog and make a beeline to the pound at our clinic! Needless-to-say, the verbal wrath of that lady descended upon the drunkard and then the town council. The bounty for taking in a "stray" was discontinued shortly after that incident!

One summer day, a client brought a young Quarter horse stallion to our clinic. He had sustained a nasty wire cut on his right front leg. I soon learned that he was a rather spoiled horse; he would try to bite a person, strike a person with a front leg and jump around when I tried to examine the wire cut.

At this point in time tranquilizers, sedation, pain killer drugs such a Xylazine, Ketamine, detomidine, butorphanol were not available for veterinarians. I resorted to applying a lip twitch on him for restraint while I treated the wire cut. It was obvious that the owner would not be able to manage follow up bandaging so I decided to hospitalize the horse for a while.

The young stallion was put in a stall in our clinic; he was obviously very ticked off with being twitched!

Later that day I had a farm call out to some cattle who had broken into an old wood bin full of wheat. When I returned to the clinic it was after 6 o'clock and I had a meeting to attend at 7. In my rush, I had unloaded a cardboard box that had about 20 packages of Oxaplus powder in it and I had just left the box on the counter in the large animal area.

During the night, the horse cleverly reached over the top of the pen gate and with his muzzle and mouth, he had slid back the bolt on the gate!

Loose in the large animal area of the clinic, he knocked carry cases and supplies off the cupboard shelves. Then in obvious spiteful glee, he bit open the packages of Oxaplus and shaking his head and neck, spread the powder all over the floor, walls and items of the large animal area! (Oxaplus powder has a taste worse than chalk so he was not biting open the packages because he was hungry!)

Next morning, I swear that he had a smirk on his face as he stood in the now white dusted large animal area of our clinic! His revenge for my twitching him the day before.

It is humbling to consider that for all of our modern medicines and equipment, nature has provided mankind with a very powerful healer: T.L.C. (tender loving care).

A client once brought an Arabian filly to our clinic; the horse's right front leg was literally dangling free at the fetlock joint. The owners thought she had got her leg wedged between angle iron braces of an old swather and then panicked. There was literally just skin holding the bottom of her leg to the rest of the leg.

"Do whatever you can", the owner said, "she's my daughter's horse". At the time synthetic fiberglass cast material had just

MORE PRACTICE REFLECTIONS

become available: lighter and much more waterproof than the old plaster cast material that we used in the past. I applied a fiberglass cast to the horse's leg and hospitalized her at our clinic. She also had treatment with antibiotics to prevent infection and pain killers for the first week. The beauty of the fiber cast was that I could cut a "small inspection window" into the cast. As time went on, radiographs (x-ray films) revealed that the bone was healing and that there was no apparent infection.

She was kept in a small stall at our clinic for one of the greatest problems for attempts to get a broken leg in a horse to heal is the fact that the horse will attempt too much weight bearing on the affected leg.

At the eight-week mark, radiographs confirmed that there was sufficient healing of the bone. However, a problem developed; the horse stopped eating and just seemed to want to lie down all the time. I could not determine a medical cause for her to have stopped eating. It seemed like she was just depressed and had given up. Drugs to enhance her appetite failed to give a response.

Totally frustrated, I came to the conclusion that it was time to send the horse home and maybe a change was all she needed.

For the first few days at home, the horse was lying down most of the time. For many years a popular chocolate bar was Peppermint Patty. The daughter spent days stroking the horse's head and feeding Peppermint Patty bars to the horse. Without any drugs or other medications, the horse perked up, developed a bright attitude and according to the owner, never looked back. This was one of the most powerful demonstrations of TLC to me!

RE: Wainwright Vet. Clinic
1301 10a St.
Wainwright, Alta.

Box 231
Killam, Alta
Sept. 20 1976

Dear Dr.s & staff;

    I thought you would be interested in finding out how Kelly is doing, so I am enclosing a picture of her taken this month. Her leg has healed much better than I thought it ever would, and her limp varies day to day from very slight to none at all! The fetlock is calcified and a degree of ringbone is still developing, but with corrective trimming, her hoof has grown out normally, and she can lead the head of horses across the pasture at full gallop with no problem at all.

    If you're ever in the area you are welcome to drop in and see how she's doing.

Sincerely,
Elaine Pyra

P.S: We're expecting her foal in early May.

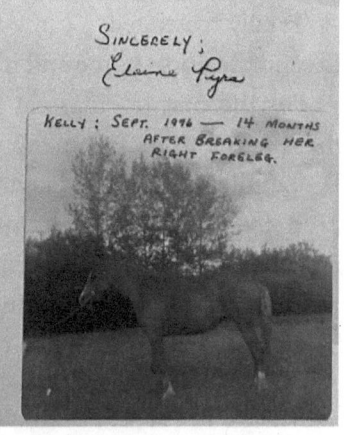

Kelly: Sept. 1976 — 14 months after breaking her right foreleg.

Thank you letter from a client

Chapter Fifteen

A FEW PERSONAL NOTES

About the second week after I started work in Wainwright, Dr. Leitch and his wife Dianne, had made arrangements one Sunday afternoon for a young lady to be at their home. They also invited me over. Keith and Dianne made generous offers of vodka. About half way through the afternoon, Keith received a call from a farmer who had a downer cow that was calving. We both left on the call out Chauvin way and left the two ladies to the vodka.

The calving case turned out to last week's case; that is the calf was very emphysematous (i.e. rotten). We performed a fetotomy to deliver the calf in pieces, both of us took turns at the fetotomy. Although wearing rubber obstetrical suits and plastic sleeves we invariably had leaks in the plastic sleeves and our arms came into contact with stinky uterine fluids. Even with a lot of scrubbing, the distinctive smell of the rotting fluid sticks with one's skin!

I had to drive the girl back home. It was a very cold January day and I had the car heater running. Evidently as stinky rotten as I smelt even with my "good looks", I didn't leave much impression on her! I often envied some of my classmates who were married before they became veterinarians.

Keith and Dianne were quite adept at providing me with names (even phone numbers) of young Wainwright girls. I met a number of them for a coffee or a movie, again with my "good looks" and unlimited charm, most meetings were once only! One of the young ladies was Eileen Killoran. She was the daughter of the Killoran family who ran a dairy farm two miles north of Wainwright. I think she took pity on me as she agreed to more dates in the future months. We attended the Gooseberry Lake rodeo and her parents had asked me for supper that day. Having over-stayed a bit at the rodeo, I was rushing to get back to Wainwright in time for the supper. I got a speeding ticket! Eileen did not say anything then but after we were married, she constantly has questions about our "altitude" when I'm driving. Little did I know that I would acquire a "co-pilot" when I was driving after I married her!

We were married on May 27, 1972; both of us had arranged for holidays for three weeks from work. For our honeymoon we went to Europe and landed in Paris. We did the usual tourist things: Eiffel Tower, Notre Dame Cathedral, the Louvre, etc. I left with a somewhat muted impression, not speaking French I soon found out that shopkeepers, clerks, etc. would try to cheat a person on monetary transactions.

We next travelled to Spain by train. Our first destination was Madrid where we spent a few days. Yes, we did attend a bull fight; we were told that it was the tourists who were keeping the bull fight tradition alive in Spain. However, there was a bull turned out that wouldn't fight; many in the crowd who I thought were Spaniards started to boo loudly and wave white handkerchiefs… ..I thought that they were going to riot!

Our next stop was Barcelona. We stayed at the Telestar Hotel. This hotel was constructed to have wing blocks of rooms leading

A FEW PERSONAL NOTES

off from an open central corridor where sewer and water line mains served each wing. We had an end-room, the bathroom was next to the open corridor; the bathrooms of the other end rooms of each wing also faced the open corridor.

Eileen went to the bathroom and moments later came out shrieking "there's a man out there"! The bathrooms each had a window with shutters and them when the shutters were open, one could see across the open corridor to open shuttered windows of the bathroom of the opposite wing. I knew then that I would have to work hard at our marriage as I wasn't sure of the context in which she screamed "there's a man out there"!

After Barcelona we spent a few days at Tossa de Mar, on the coast of the Mediterranean Sea. Very enjoyable, very reasonable lodging and meals and great weather.

Next we travelled by train to Zurich, Switzerland for a couple days, beautiful country.

Eileen's sister Kathleen and her husband Rick Belkie, lived near Baden-Baden, Germany. Rick served in the Canadian Army and was stationed with Canadian and American soldiers at the Lahr, Germany NATO base. When we arrived in Germany, a German official was checking our passports. He recognized my name (Schatz) as German and started speaking to me in German. Embarrassed, I had to convey to him that I didn't speak German.

We spent about one week in Germany with Rick and Kathleen. This was still the era of the Cold War and when Rick drove us around, it was somewhat comical. Rick said that there were spies everywhere and sure enough literally behind every tree, one could see a partially hidden man with binoculars!

Rick drove us to Frankfurt for a flight to Paris as our return flight to Canada was from Paris. The Orly Massacre had occurred at the Orly Airport during our stay in Europe; before our flight departed, one didn't feel safe scratching one's face or making any sudden move. Soldiers and police with sub-machine guns were everywhere and the atmosphere was extremely tense.

Our first home was an old farmhouse on an acreage that just adjoined the northwest corner of the town of Wainwright limits. The house had two additions made to it and mostly a dirt basement. The bedroom floor was sinking towards the center. I had to put cedar shingles under the front of our dresser to keep the drawers from sliding out on their own.

Kerry-Ann was born on October 5, 1973 and perhaps due to poor planning, Travis was born two years later exactly on October 5, 1975. The twins, Lanny and Jason were our surprise package, born on July 21, 1978. Eileen had dreamt about having twins, her doctor said no (I think her doctor was more excited than we were in the delivery room)!

Eileen continued working as a dental assistant after we were married and for awhile after Kerry was born. The spring of 1973 was extremely busy as the exotic cattle boom was still on; there were days when I might see Eileen driving to work and wave to her as I was driving out to a country call. It was also quite an experience for Eileen to handle all of the farmers' vet calls. She was amazed how different dental practice was from veterinary practice.

After the bulk of the calving season work was finished, in June of 1973, Eileen and I took a "decompression" holiday to the Hawaiian Islands. The scenery and some of the tourist attractions were amazing but I found some of the "American commercialization" a bit of a put off.

On the island of Maui, I rented a car and we drove the back roads; away from all the fancy tourist sites, we were astounded at the poverty of some of the native people in the back country areas of Maui. In one small village, there was a movie theatre which was playing the newly released movie, the Posidean Adventure. We attended this movie with a crowd of the locals; about halfway

A FEW PERSONAL NOTES

through the movie, the projector broke down. It was several years later back in Canada before we were able to watch that movie through to the end. Of note in 2023, that village area of Maui was burned down, apparently deliberate to free up more land for the tourist development.

Over the following years, with our family, we made trips during the summer to visit family as well as camping trips to Dillberry Lake, Long Lake, Muriel Lake, Moose Lake, Jasper National Park, Waterton Park and Sylvan Lake.

In 1982, one of the companies from which we purchased veterinary drugs and products, had an "air miles type" promotion based on volume of purchases. The tickets were for Jamaica, where a joint Canadian/Caribbean Veterinary conference was being held in the fall of 1982. By a "pooling" arrangement with one of our neighboring colleagues, enough points were obtained so that Eileen, the four kids and myself were able to go to Jamaica….. Eileen had talked to the kids at great length about tanning versus sunburn in a hot climate.

When the airplane landed in Montego Bay, Jamaica, as we disembarked, Travis spotted a very dark native Jamaican and yelled out in a loud voice "Mom, I'm going to turn that black"? Interestingly, Dr. Pearce Louisey who had a small animal practice in Calgary, was out on the beach with us one day. He was originally from one of the Caribbean Islands and quite dark skinned. After a few minutes on the beach as we were putting shirts back on Dr. Louisey said "I have to get a shirt too, you know Art, after being away from a lot of sun, I will burn as bad as you"!

In 1985, the Canadian Veterinary Conference was hosted in Penticton, B.C. On our trip there, we stopped in Jasper National Park. First night was marked by one of the twins dousing Eileen's feet with profuse diarrhea. Next day, while out on a boat tour on the lake, the other twin doused me with vomit. On the rest of the trip to Penticton, the killer flu also hit Kerry, Travis and Eileen. At the conference we met Dr. Robert Miller from California; he was a famous veterinary cartoonist and he drew a cartoon animal for each of our kids.

On our trip back to Alberta, we stopped at Summerland, B.C. where my former school teacher, Iris Coffman and her husband Norval (former 4-H club leader) had retired. Sadly Iris gave us news of her on-going battle with cancer. Our next stop on the way back was at Cowley, Alberta where my uncle Martin Schatz farmed; he was quite famous for his folk carvings of wood whirl-a-jigs, a couple of which are displayed in the Glenbow Museum in Calgary.

Next stop was to Bow Island to visit my Mom and Dad, brothers and their families. Back on afterwards to Wainwright for my niece Jennifer's wedding at which the twins were the ring bearers.

In 1980 we built a new home on our acreage, it was in the shape of a "T", the main portion had the bedrooms. Major design fault: the kids bedrooms faced to the south where a drive-in movie theatre was located. In later years, they admitted to us that they pretended to be asleep; waited until Eileen and I were asleep, then got up, opened the curtains and evidently could watch movies. They also admitted that most of the movies could not be rated as family!

At Wainwright Kerry and Travis were members of the 4-H Beef and 4-H Light Horse Clubs. I served as leader of the Greenshields 4-H Beef Club for three years. One year we added a dairy heifer project for a few kids. When we moved to Fairview, the kids continued in 4-H projects and I served a couple years as leader of the Fairview 4-H Beef Club.

Over the years, our family had many dogs, cats, rabbits, chickens, turkeys, a few horses and lots of cattle. As a veterinarian, one is supposed to be a "Superhero" for one's kids. Mentally and emotionally I went through some of the toughest times when we lost a favourite pet, death of one of our own animals, or when the time had come to send one of our animals over the rainbow bridge.

In addition to the risk of acquiring zoonotic infections, veterinarians also have the risk of physical injury. A client once brought in a 2800 pound Shorthorn/Simmental bull for hoof trimming. As we were in the process of putting him onto a large animal tilt table, he nailed me in my right knee and I fell to the clinic floor. I managed to get myself up and complete the hoof trim. The cruciate ligaments in my right knee had been ruptured; I had surgical repair done at the Misercordia hospital and a plaster cast applied for a while. Once while out pregnancy testing cows, a heavy drop gate with angle iron trim came down on the left foot. I had broken metatarsal bones; I bought a pair of lace work boots. With the left boot laced up very tight, I was able to continue pregnancy testing work that fall.

The complications of arthritis in the left foot and right knee developed in the years following those injuries. I had a number of cortisone injections over time in the left ankle joint and the right knee. The injections did help the pain initially but later on the effect was minimal.

In 2019, I was booked to have surgery to fuse the tarsal joint in my left ankle. With the advent of the COVID outbreak, the surgery was delayed, and I think over the next three years the ankle joint fused on its own (anyway it stopped bothering me). Meanwhile, my right knee was unstable and painful. March 12 of 2024, I finally had right knee replacement surgery and as of this writing, that knee now feels better than it has in years!

There was a period of about three years in which Fairview College's Agriculture program became involved in an exchange program with agriculture colleges in Russia. This was the time when Gorbachev was President of Russia, and he was attempting to open Russia up to the rest of the world.

In 1992, I was selected (along with two other college instructors and two AHT students) to participate in a three-week trip to Russia. First leg of our trip took us to Kiev by plane; the real eye opening was that there were people standing in the aisle of the Aeroflot plane during flight! Upon arrival in Kiev, my suitcase was missing (it showed up mysteriously at the Grande Prairie airport one month after I was back in Canada)! I had a small backpack carry-on with an extra shirt, pants and pair of gaunchies.

We only had one day in Kiev before we left by train to go to Stavropol in southwestern Russia. It was at this time that Gorbachev gave the Ukraine back its self-control. Although we didn't speak Ukrainian there was an obvious sense of optimism and joy among the people of Kiev with dancing in the streets. There was one area where the dancing people had taken off all of their clothes in their celebration! (I feel a lot of sadness for the Ukrainian people in light of the current Russian-Ukrainian war.)

The train was our first inclination that in terms of development the "clock had stopped" about 30 years ago in the Communist states. We had been assigned an interpreter upon arrival and he accompanied us to Stavropol.

In Stavropol we were given rooms in a student's residence associated with a university in that city. The toilet and plumbing in my room were ancient and there was no hot water. I had the impression that under Communism no one "gave a shit" as there was no pride in workmanship. A hot water pipe lead to a radiator heater that was half-way across a doorway as the installer couldn't be bothered to shorten the pipe. Someone had started to paint the trim around a door but evidently stopped and left at one point, never to complete the job.

Initially our reception at the university seemed very frosty for two reasons. Number one – a group of Russian students was supposed to have come to Fairview College before our trip to Russia. At that time there was a high rate of tuberculosis[19] in Russia and

A FEW PERSONAL NOTES

testing for T.B. was required before their trip to Canada. The Russians had not met the health requirements and their exchange group was denied entry to Canada. Again, there was the language barrier, but it was obvious that the Russians were not happy to host us. Number two – an unfortunate side effect of Gorbachev's reforms was devaluation of the Russian ruble, and I got the sense that "money was tight" for them and to host us was a burden. However, over the course of our visit a high level of hospitality developed.

The University of Stavropol had a veterinary college as well as an agriculture college. The Rector (President) of the university was a veterinarian and he had a son who was also a veterinarian. I enjoyed touring their veterinary college as they had very extensive numbers of skeletons, assorted bones and other specimens for anatomy and pathology classes. I had the impression that their clinical medicine was behind North America; for example, they had no vaccines for small animals. In one of their labs, the professor was demonstrating the use of xylazine on a dog…..xylazine had just become available to them in Russia. We had that drug available for veterinary use for many years previously in Canada.

The young veterinarian had just received his master's degree. His paper was on nitrate poisoning, and this was regarded as a new discovery. In North America the pathogenesis of a nitrate poisoning in cattle had been known for years. Again, this was an example of the "time clock stopping" because the Communists so severely restricted contact with the west and the exchange of knowledge was almost zero.

Our visit included visits to a couple of communal farms, slaughter-house, sheep ranch, etc. Most of these visits left me rather miffed as it was obvious that there was a level of "cover up" and we were limited as to what we were allowed to observe. President Mikhail Gorbachev was trying to establish private farming and it seemed to me that the concept was difficult for

Russian farmers to adopt. While touring the communal farm, there were again many signs of a "don't give a shit" worker attitude: a load of bricks was dumped out of a truck box in a hurry with about half of the bricks broken. I had the impression that Communism did create work but many of the jobs were examples of inefficiency; example there was a dedicated person to put the pin in the drawbar of a tractor and that appeared to be his work for the day until the cultivator was unhooked from the tractor at the end of the day.

I visited a couple of stores in Stavropol to buy a few clothes since my suitcase had gone A.W.O.L. It was an eye opener to observe that their shops were literally empty of stock. After a few days I learned of an area where there was a black market for western goods. Evidently western clothes, radios, watches were brought in by car to sell at a black market. I was able to purchase some clothing there. One morning, I observed a long line up by a grocery store, people had heard that after many days wait, a shipment of butter had come into the state-owned store.

Another amusing observation was that most of their cars on the road appeared to be very well used old Ladas. It seemed like there was some kind of problem getting tires as most of the Ladas had bald tires. Indeed, everywhere someone was stopped on the side of the road, changing a flat tire. Also evident were many cars on the side of the road with apparent mechanical breakdowns. On our field trips I would often notice a vehicle on the side of the road in the morning and on the return trip the vehicle had been stripped down for parts. This was the Russian struggle at that time.

One of our tours was out to a sheep ranch to the east of Stavropol, in the Chechnya region, we had to pass through several check points with a number of armed soldiers and an army tank at each check point. With Gorbachev's reforms, many of the countries in the U.S.S.R. were trying to break away and have their

A FEW PERSONAL NOTES

own governments. There had been armed revolts in Chechnya during that era of time.

We visited the Caucasus mountains region which was a resort like area of Russia. There was an "arts" area with many painters, crafts people displaying and selling their works. I purchased a painting and a metal work piece of art. There were a number of apartment like complex buildings in the Caucasus, the interpreter said that they were "rest homes". I later learned that they were T.B. sanitoriums built in the favorable climate of the Caucasus.

Although the communist regime had suppressed religion for many decades after Gorbachev "opened" up Russia, there was the fact that many Russian people were very happy to now attend church services. Communism had not suppressed religion.

Russia had a high level of tuberculosis in its farm livestock and had been unsuccessful in any of their government programs to eliminate T.B. from their livestock. I contrast this to Canada where our national test and slaughter federal program has our national rate of T.B. in cattle down to about 0.01% or less today.

An observation on our tours was the presence of vendors on the side of the highway selling cuts of pork....no refrigeration evident and with farm slaughter no likely government inspection for lesions of tuberculosis. (There is a human species of T.B., but the animal T.B. species can be transmitted to humans by contact or infected meat or milk.)

In spite of the stated goal of equality for all people, it was very obvious that a "rich class" of citizens had evolved under Communism (much as in western capitalist countries). As we got to know our Russian hosts it was obvious that the Russian people were much like us once the barrier of political beliefs was scaled.

I retired from the college June 30, 2010…..the one year stint had somehow evolved into 23 years at that employment. Now I could concentrate on loosing money on my small cattle operation. For many years, I was a member of the Peace Country Beef

& Forage Association which hosted many seminars and tours for me to participate in.

During the course of our marriage, if Eileen and I had a spat, she would bring up the topic that I had a couple of aunts who were a bit "daffy". I had quite a number of aunts, uncles and cousins in Canada; Eileen only had her parents, brothers and sisters in Canada (fewer chances for a verbal counter attack at her)!

Eileen's brother John became involved with the dairy board for Canada and participated in quite a number of trade missions to various countries, one of which was Ireland. He was able to make contact with long-lost cousins in Ireland; over the years, Eileen's parents avoided saying much about any relatives in Ireland. One year, one of our nephews was getting married and a cousin from Ireland arrived to attend the wedding.

During the course of drinks at the wedding, the cousin revealed a "family secret". Eileen's grandfather on her mother's side ran a livery business in Ireland (like a taxi only horse and buggy). Reportedly one rainy day he delivered a nobleman to an Irish pub; he was instructed to wait (in the rain) for the nobleman for the return trip. When he took the nobleman home, the two got into an argument over the fare and a fight ensued. Eileen's grandfather reportedly had beaten the nobleman with a cudgeon stick. Fearing that he had killed the nobleman, Eileen's grandfather took a ship to New York, leaving behind Eileen's pregnant grandmother and two kids.

Some tracing revealed that he had gone to Montreal and remarried. I think that is known as bigamy, the family secret Eileen's Mom and Dad were too ashamed to talk about. But talk about karma, after this revelation, Eileen never got on my case about my relatives!

In 2012, Eileen and I, her two sisters and her two nieces made a trip to Ireland. In addition to touring a few tourist sites in Dublin, we travelled by train to the Sligo area of Ireland where we

A FEW PERSONAL NOTES

visited a number of Eileen's long- lost cousins. Eileen was able to view the ruins of the stone house where her father grew up and also the abandoned house where her mother grew up. Oh yes, our visit included a couple of traditional Irish bar nights.

In 2014, Eileen and I went on a bus tour of Ireland which included visits to many famous tourist sites such as Castle Rock, Bunratty Castle and yes, we kissed the Blarney Stone (I still don't have the gift of gab, it's a hoax). We toured a bit of Northern Ireland, such sites as the Titanic Memorial, Giant's Causeway and the "wall" in Belfast. At the end of the bus tour, we spent a few days visiting Eileen's cousins in the Sligo area, sadly since 2012, two of the ones we met then had passed away.

Later in the fall of 2014, my son Travis took me on a tour in Australia which was sponsored by the Peace Country Beef & Forage Association. Our tour included visits to three beef ranches, a dairy, crayfish processing plant, an abattoir and of course a number of tourist sites. That year Australia was experiencing a drought. It was interesting to compare how their farmers handled drought to the ways we handled drought in Canada. It seemed too easy to bond with the affable Australians.

Starting in 2012, my left ankle joint started to affect my walking and as the years progressed my knees also were proving to be issues. I started to wish that I had toured more than I was younger. By the spring of 2020, when I was sitting on a newborn calf to tag it, a revelation became clear; I no longer had the physical strength and mobility to be doing ranch work.

We sold Westview Ranch in 2021 and Eileen and I are currently residing in Garrison Manor in Fairview. At the time of this writing, I am recovering from right knee replacement surgery.

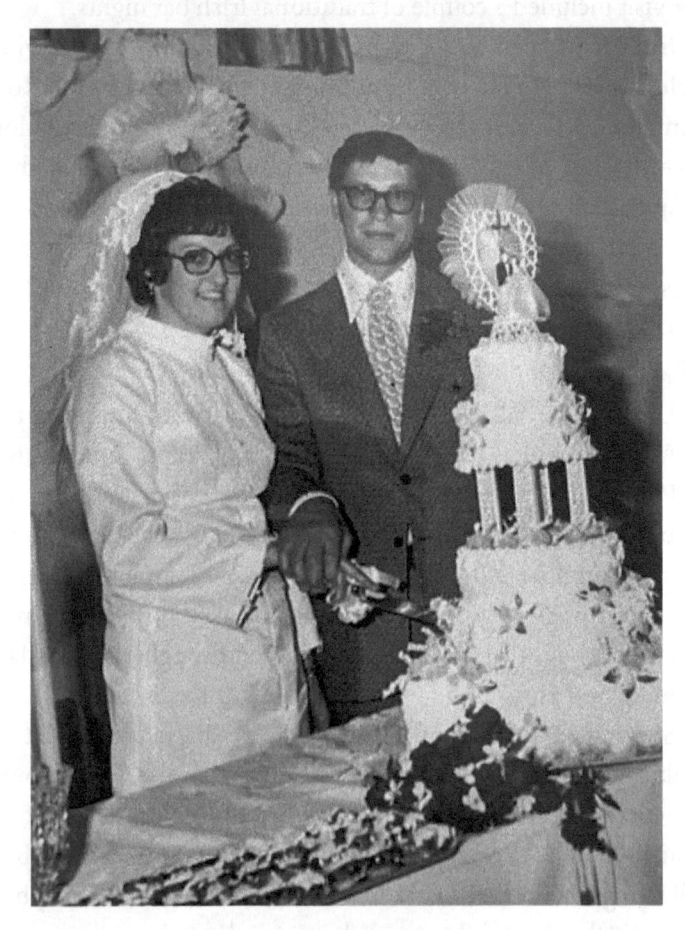

Wedding Day May 27th 1972

A FEW PERSONAL NOTES

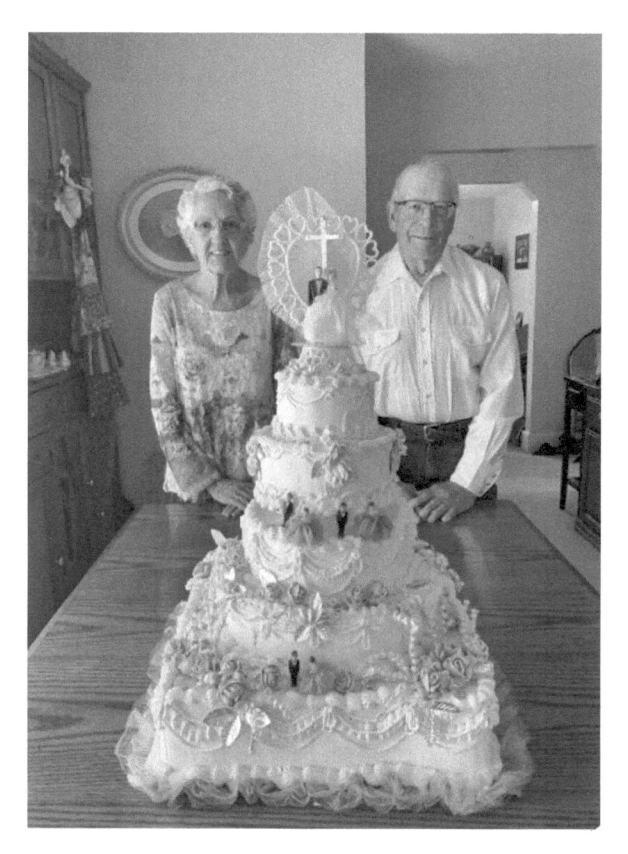

50th Anniversary. Even the model cake survived!

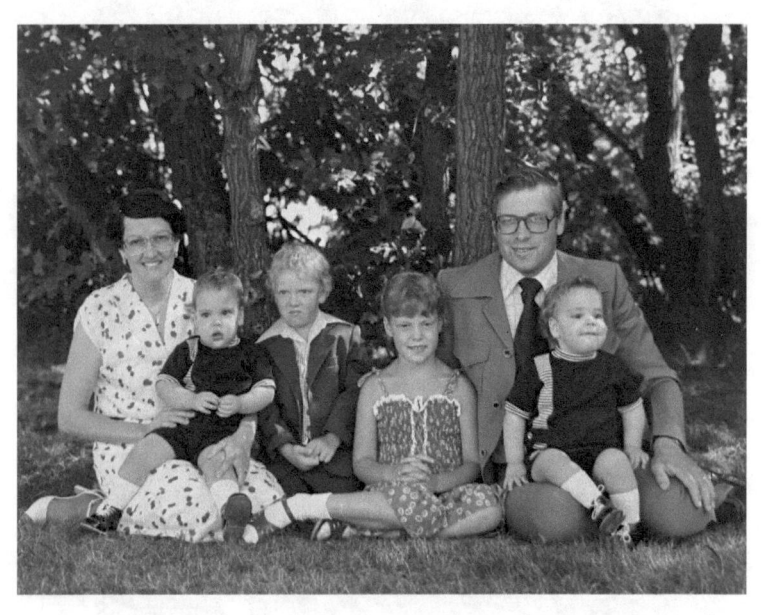

Family 1979 (left to right) Eileen, Lanny, Travis, Kerry, Art, Jason

A FEW PERSONAL NOTES

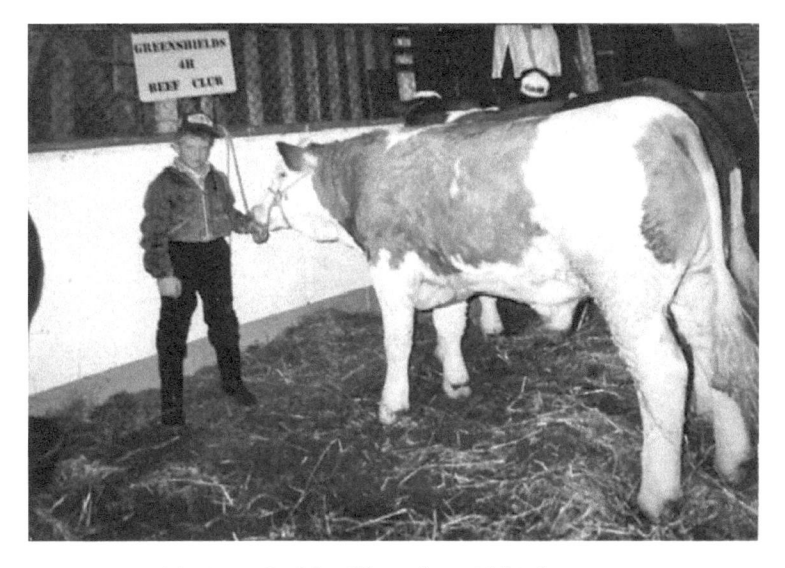

Travis as a PeeWee 4H member with his first steer

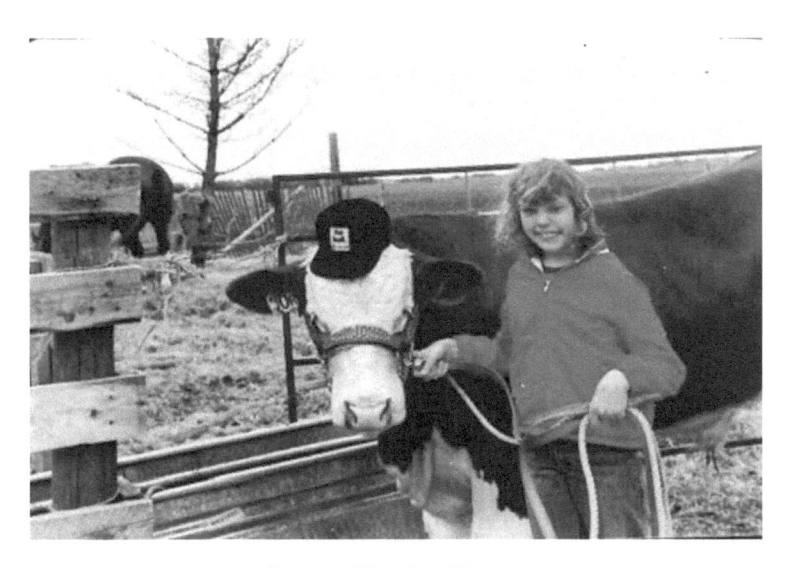

Kerry and her first 4H steer

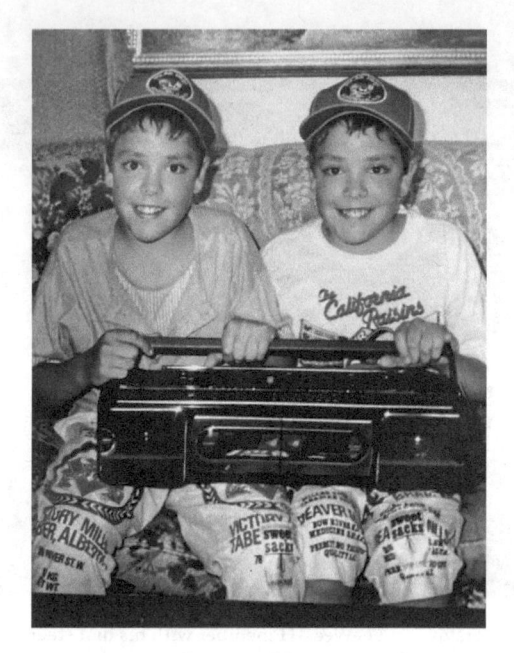

Lanny and Jason

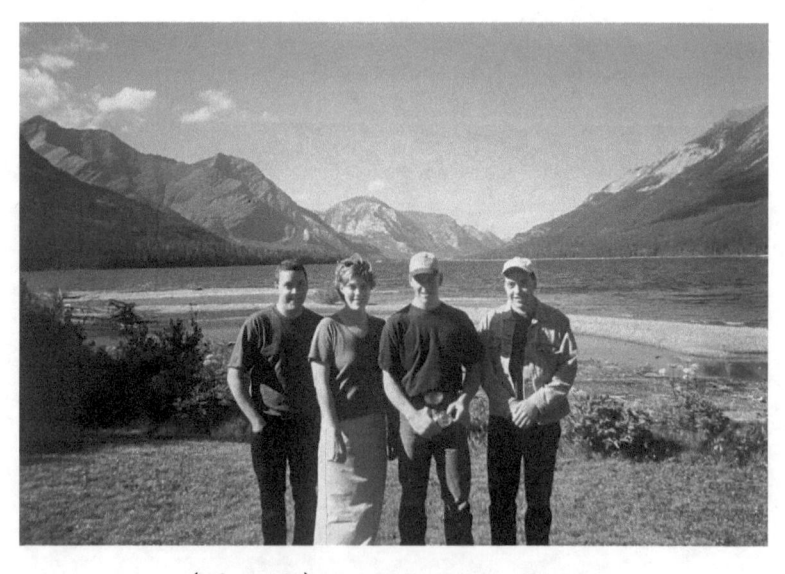

(left to right) Jason, Kerry, Travis and Lanny

Chapter Sixteen

WESTVIEW RANCH ALIAS POVERTY ACRES

When we moved to Fairview, we stayed for several months at an acreage northeast of Fairview, then for about one year at a rented college house on campus and then at a rental acreage northwest of Fairview.

In the spring of 1988, I noticed an ad for tenders for a Farm Credit sale of a property west and a bit south of Fairview. One block of the sale land was a half-section located on a point between the Hines Creek coulee and the Island Creek coulee. The farm site was once a dairy farm with a 24 foot by 72 foot barn, an older house, old garage, cattle shed, corrals and some granaries. It was run down but most of the south quarter was an open grassy area of the Hines Creek coulee with a tremendous view to the south. To the west, the west side of the Hines Creek coulee was higher than the farm east side, so there was also a nice view to the west.

We wanted to live in the country and at the time there were few rural properties for sale in the Fairview area. Somewhat mesmerized by the view and the possibilities of the Farm Credit land, we put in a bid tender for the west half of 19 81 4 W6. Our bid was later accepted....in retrospect, I think we learned why it was a Farm Credit sale: perhaps something about air currents or flow at the convergence of the two coulees but time over time, the land on the west side of the Hines Creek coulee would get a heavy rain. The rain would skip over our place and farmers on the east side of the Island Creek coulee would get the heavy rain again!

Parts of the Island Creek coulee to the east, Hines Creek coulee to the south and west were a grazing lease of about 1280 acres, the open area of my south quarter was surrounded by this grazing lease, so it all was shared with the grazing lease holders, Jack Mehlsen and Ray Nikiforuk. I was also able to obtain another Hines Creek coulee grazing lease to the northwest of my property.

There was about 176 acres of cultivated land on our half section. For a number of years I rented it out on a crop share basis to neighboring farmers. In later years I had it seeded down to alfalfa and meadow brome grass. With the adjacent grazing leases, it seemed more sense to run a small cattle ranch hence Westview Ranch alias Poverty Acres came to be!

Another reality check after purchase of the property, the existing house was located right beside a dam (dugout) and as we inspected the dirt basement, we observed several burnt out sump pumps. There was a cistern for hauled in drinking water but the walls appeared cracked!

We made a decision to build a new house to the south on bit of a knoll. The old house was sold and moved off. In August of 1990, we moved into our new home....at last, a permanent home in the Fairview area.

Another feature to the property was the location of four natural gas wells and a compressor station owned at the time by Anderson Exploration. In later years with the advent of directional drilling technology, another five gas wells would be drilled into areas of the Hines Creek coulee.

I put a new metal roof on the barn, cattle shed and the granaries. There had been two or three previous owners since the time of the dairy farm there so the interior had been converted into horse box stalls. The lower wall of the south side was rotted out as someone had not cleaned out manure often enough. I rebuilt that south wall. Next project I completed was to sheet the loft floor.

October of 1992, we had a barn fire and the barn burned completely down. The north side of the barn had a small lean-to addition (one time milk room probably); we used this as a tack room so saddles, bridles, halters, etc. were lost. I had just purchased and stacked about 1200 square hay bales in the barn, perhaps there was a bale that overheated….not sure of the cause of the fire though. Losing the barn was very traumatic for our family. I can't imagine the emotional trauma of losing a house to fire!

The northwest quarter section had a small coulee draw cutting off the northeast portion of that quarter. At one time someone had built a fence down and up that small coulee draw to fence off that corner as a small holding pasture. Again, when I took over the place, that fence was in a sad state of repair; fallen trees, overgrowth, down and broken barb wire. I undertook the task of resurrecting and rebuilding that fence, again in my naivety as a guy from flat southern Alberta, it turned out to be a very grueling task. There was one area where the slope was so steep that one could barely stand let alone balance to swing a mallet to pound a fence post! I had about an 80- pound pipe hand post pounder with side handles welded up. It did work somewhat better than a mallet on the rock-hard coulee hill.

Our kids were in 4-H with steer, heifer and horse projects. The heifers were the start of a small herd of cows. Similar to a schoolteacher, as an instructor I had the summer months off. A sane person would have gone travelling or to a beach, but no, I had to undertake fencing as summer "rest and relaxation"!

I guess the land and the cattle were a lifestyle decision for me. As the years went by I probably should have expanded to more land to justify for more cattle (or vice versa) to have more of a viable economic unit. As Einstein said, "the definition of stupidity is to do the same thing over and over again with the same results". Yup! I do use the excuse that due to my health issues, I held back on enlarging my small cattle operation. Guess that I had the luxury of my college salary to subsidize the cattle.

Mother Nature doles out the weather in cycles in my experience, sometimes "wet years" with ample rainfall and sometimes dry years with virtually no rain. I found out that in a dry year the length of time of grazing in the coulee lease was very short. The cattle had to be moved back to the tame hay/pasture land which I wanted to save for fall grazing. That led to buying more hay than anticipated or selling off some of the herd.

Due to our friendship with John Milne, one of the original importers of the Gelbvieh breed of cattle, we had purchased Gelbvieh 4-H heifers from John; this lead to the gradual build up of our Gelbvieh herd. We had a number of purebred Gelbvieh and were selling yearling bulls. BSE was diagnosed in cattle in Canada in May of 2003 and the price of cattle fell to rock bottom. That year we were selling the Gelbvieh yearling bulls for $2,000 each, at the time when BSE (Bovine Spongiform Encephalopathy) (Mad Cow Disease) hit, we had three left to sell. No market for them as the BSE shut down evolved so we shipped them for slaughter. We netted about $166 each for those three bulls.

The effect of BSE[20] was a drastic reduction in the Canadian cattle herd over the next few years, ours included. Along with the BSE downturn, we also faced some successive drought years. Tough times.

A couple that we were friends with and I hit upon the plan to have some of our cattle slaughtered, the meat cut and wrapped and we would take loaded deep freezers in a trailer up to Hay River and Yellowknife in the Northwest Territories for sale there. We could get a better price for our cattle (even after the long- haul drive) this way than we could at local markets. The plan was successful for a while but then the grocery stores in the Territories started to squawk about us to their government. We were given an order to cease. The stores in the north have a very captive market and they didn't like our miniscule competition.

As a note, once there were three local abattoirs within about 12 miles of Fairview, they are now shut down, partly due to government regulations and red tape and the effects of the major meat packing plants at Brooks and High River. This trend in the demise of many local abattoirs was seen throughout Alberta.

The ripple effects of BSE over the years also lead to fewer cattle truckers, closure of some auction markets and yes, it severely affected many veterinary practices.

For many years, the Alberta government has sponsored an Environmental Farm Plan Program. Farmers and ranchers complete an assessment of their operation as to corral drainage of manure runoff, location of wells, dugouts, storage practices for farm chemicals and commercial fertilizers, etc. The objective is to make farm/ranch operations more environmentally friendly. Once an environmental farm plan was completed, there were government grant programs to help the owner make improvements such as moving corrals to a better location.

There were corrals by the old barn and cattle shed however, these were located right on top of the south side of a small coulee draw; this draw led eventually to the Island Creek coulee and then eventually to the Peace River. I applied for and was successful for a grant to relocate the corrals on our property to an area east and south of our new house. Any corral drainage would not go into the coulee from this new site. Constructing the new corrals/handling facilities was a major fall/winter project for me one year, I sure pounded a lot of spike nails!

The previous owner had some old holding/sorting pens by a very dilapidated runway chute. A bit of karma perhaps, but when I was in practice, there were situations where I was on a farm pregnancy testing cows and part of the owner's corral was a thin half-broken sheet of plywood that the cows busted through. Next year, same farm, same half busted sheet of plywood. I have to confess that it was several years before I rebuilt the cattle handling facilities on my place. It would be a very revealing and humbling experience for every large animal veterinarian to experience owning and maintaining their own cattle operation before going out on farm calls and muttering about some farmer's set up!

Likewise, it is very humbling for a veterinarian to own his own livestock: they still seem to get sick, have calving problems and prolapses. Of course, these problems usually occurred at night or when I was at work at the college!

After I retired from the college, when there was a problem with the cattle, my wife would remind me that I really wasn't "semi-retired" but that I was "semi-stunned". She said "you spent years and years in practice getting crapped on, stepped on, crushed, kicked, smashed and run over"! "And you still keep cattle now"?

As I mentioned previously, living in the country and having the cattle was for me a bit of a lifestyle choice. The grazing lease in the Hines Creek coulee had areas where the sides of the coulee had slumped (a slide), leaving a couple area that were in essence sloughs on the side of the long coulee hill. When I was fencing in those areas, my rest breaks would involve time just spent watching beavers, geese and ducks that inhabited those sloughs. There were many chipmunks, squirrels, deer, moose and the occasional elk to observe. Black bears also travelled the coulee. Once I heard the cry of a cougar nearby, didn't see it but a neighbor who was combining did see it. I never had any cattle losses due to bear or cougar in all the years that I ran cattle in those coulees.

In southern Alberta where I grew up, we did not have any moose in that area, only deer and pronghorn antelope. I confess to a learning curve in regards to moose. One winter we had a lot of heavy snowfalls; I had the Municipal District snowplow come into the yard and plow out the laneway, circular turn around in front of the house and garage, leaving high steep banks of snow on each side of the road. I was shoveling snow off the front steps when I heard Turk, our young Anatolian Shepherd dog, barking continuously at the area where we had a garden spot. Carrying the snow shovel, I walked down to where he was, still barking vigorously. Among some tame Saskatoon tree bushes, there was a large bull moose, happily stripping the bark off of the tree branches.

I waved the snow shovel at him and yelled out a suggestion to him to the effect that he should "go forth and procreate"! In a flash, he bounded over the snow bank onto the laneway and charged me. I only a moment to hold the snow shovel out in front of me (boy do I ever remember the look in his yellow eyes) and he hit the snow shovel with his head, bowling me over flat on my back. I vividly remember the hoof of one of his hindlegs coming down right beside my face as he leapt over me! Fortunately, he kept running with Turk running and barking at his side as if to say, some fun let's play.

Turk was with us for 10 years; he developed a routine (I think natural for an Anatolian Shepherd) to patrol about a two-mile radius around our farm. I recall one day, he spotted a young coyote, snuck out using the round bale stack as a cover, then ambushed the coyote. I was about 700 feet away, but I could still hear the coyote's bones snapping as Turk finished the coyote off.

However, as a guard dog we found that he did not have a "people personality" as with our Golden Retrievers.

We had a spell of years in which we had Louisiana Catahoula as our farm dogs. Travis had bought into the hype that they would go down into the coulee and bay, causing the cattle to come up to the top of the coulee. However, this did not work out as they seemed more adept at baying outside of our house in the middle of the night!

For the first number of years, I bought hay for our cattle operation with the thought that I couldn't justify a line of new haying equipment for the size of our cattle herd. Someone convinced me that I could make do with used equipment, so I went through years with a used Heston round baler, then an old New Holland 851 and then an old John Deere 525. Another learning curve as I'm not a good mechanic. Some people had a square baler, some people a round baler; most times I think that I had a "swear baler"!

I vividly recall one incident while baling alfalfa hay. Looking back as I dumped a finished bale out on the John Deere baler. I noticed some black smoke. I left the tailgate of the baler up and ran back to have a look. Sure enough there was a hot, burnt out bearing on the end of one of the rollers. Fearing that the baler belts and loose alfalfa leaves would catch on fire, I frantically started to kick the ground to be able to pick up loose dirt to throw on the hot bearing.

When I felt that it was under control, I exhaustedly staggered around to the front of the baler. Wiping the sweat off of my forehead with my right arm, I rested against the LARGE ROUND SILVER FIRE EXTINGUISHER! Arrgh! As I have related before, I don't think that I could even be accused of intelligence!

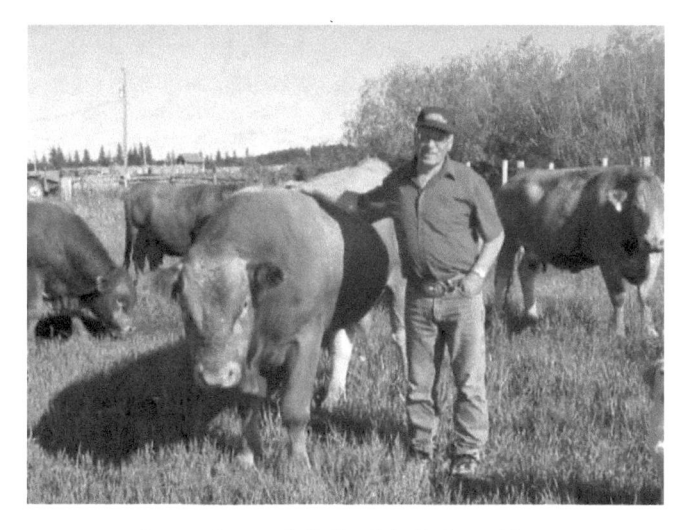

Outstanding with Gelbvieh bull, Super Mario

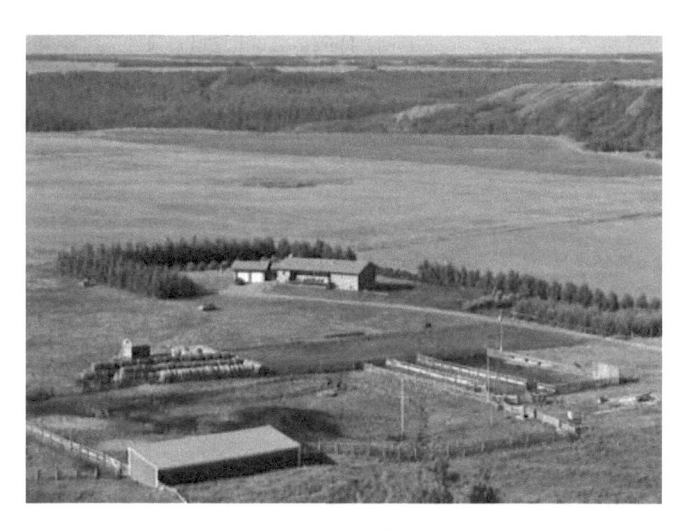

Westview Ranch 1996

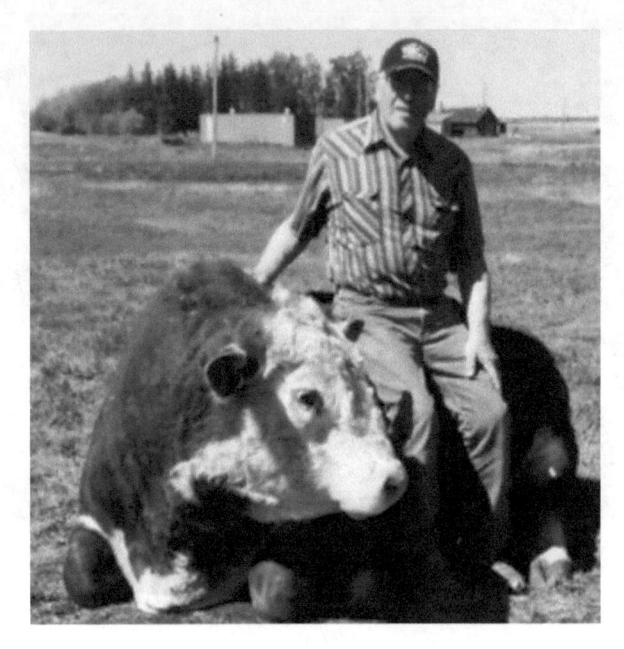

Lazing around with Hereford bull, Bullseye

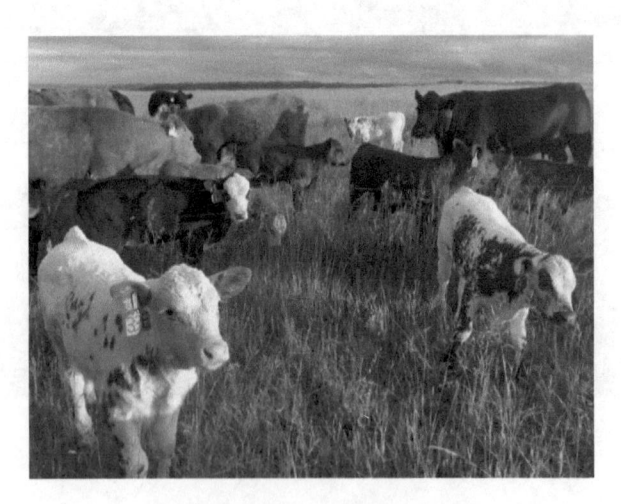

Crossbred cattle on Westview Ranch

Chapter Seventeen

PROFESSIONAL GOVERNANCE

In the 1970's, I served a term on the Council of the Alberta Veterinary Medical Association. One of our areas of jurisdiction was dealing with complaints from the public against members of the Association. These complaints varied from the frivolous to those of a very serious if not illegal nature.

As professionals, veterinarians are given the right to a rather independent level of self-governing and self-policing as laid out in the Veterinary Profession Act[11], provincial legislation of Alberta. There were several inadequacies of the Act at that time and as Council we were lobbying the provincial government to amend parts of the Act. (It took several years for the Act to be amended.)

At that time, as Council, we assessed the complaint, then if warranted we investigated the complaint and then we made a ruling on the complaint.

Due to human nature, I think every profession or trade is subject to having a few bad actors, our veterinary profession included. For example, one of the cases we dealt with was that of a registered Black Labrador dog that had been hit by a car. The dog was limping on one hindleg. The owner took this dog to a veterinarian for examination; this veterinarian showed the owner radiographs (x-ray pictures) to the effect that the dog had a broken femur bone which would require a stainless- steel pin be placed down the center of the bone to hold the broken pieces together until the bone healed. The owner agreed to and paid for that orthopedic surgery and the dog was later discharged with skin sutures on the side of its hindleg.

The dog was returned a number of days later for suture removal as is the standard and then the dog was to be returned in a few weeks for follow-up radiographs to see if the bone was healed satisfactorily and if the steel pin could be removed (standard practice).

In the following weeks, the owner moved to another location and took his dog to the veterinary practice in that area. When the second veterinarian radiographed the dog, there was no steel pin and the femur had never been broken! The owner filed a complaint against the first veterinarian to our Council.

As it was a registered dog, there was an ear tattoo noted in the first veterinarian's case record, this tattoo matched with the owners. We made the judgement that the first veterinarian was guilty of a fraud and made the judgement to strip him of his right to practice. He appealed our decision in the court system of Alberta (turned out he had more money in his bank coffers for legal fees than all of our Veterinary Association had at that time)!

As Council of the Alberta Veterinary Medical Association, we lost his appeal; the judge ruled that we as Council had acted as the investigating body (i.e. police) and as judge and jury! This was not how the court system was supposed to function but due to the oversights in the provincial legislation, we had acted according to the Act! Justice is blind but not immune to technicalities!

At present time, (after frustrating years our Veterinary Professionals Act was finally amended by the provincial government) a complaint against a veterinarian is investigated by an appointed investigator. The report of the investigation is reported to a Complaint Review Committee; this committee may dismiss the case due to insufficient evidence or due to the complaint as being judged frivolous. If there is deemed to be merit to the complaint a decision is made for the veterinarian to appear before a Hearing Tribunal.

At a formal hearing with the veterinarian, the Hearing Tribunal may make a range of decisions varying from absolution to the removal of the veterinarian's right to practice. Monetary fines and legal costs are sometimes assessed, sometimes written reprimand, changes to protocols or sometimes required continuing education requests are mandated.

The whole complaints process is managed by a Complaints Director, a hired position of the Alberta Veterinary Medical Association. In 2023, 35 members were subject of a complaint, this represents 0.82% of 4267 registered members. I do feel that the system is a great improvement from the time of my involvement on Council and I feel our profession does make a sincere effort to address the public concerns.

My oldest brother fought a long difficult battle with multiple sclerosis (MS). At one point one of his daughters convinced a lawyer to disclosure of the contents of a will of my brothers even though my brother was still alive. I filed a complaint with the Law Society of Alberta (governing body for the legal profession in Alberta). My first complaint to the Law Society was shrugged off but I filed the complaint again. The Law Society did call a formal hearing for that lawyer. He was given a reprimand, fined $500 for his misdemeanor and banned from ever receiving the designation of Queen's Council. I present this story to serve as a contrast between legal complaints and veterinary complaints in Alberta; it seems as if the veterinary profession is subject to more severe disciplinary action with fines sometimes in the thousands of dollars.

At the time of my first year in practice, any form of advertising our services was forbidden by our veterinary association. A classmate of mine was reprimanded for handing out business cards with his phone number when he started his practice. We could have our clinic listed in a phone book but we were essentially limited to "word of mouth" by one client to another to build our practice. The profession's ethics rules have changed vastly in the past 55 years, and I am astounded by the scope of advertising that is now permitted for today's practicing veterinarians.

Chapter Eighteen

THOUGHTS: FUTURE OF THE VETERINARY PROFESSION

It is said that some people who have suffered abuse or a bad experience can blot it from their memory. I wish that I had that ability; the reader may have gotten the impression from reading this book that my veterinary practice career was nothing but disasters. There were certainly many rewarding and successful cases however in my mind I tend to still fret over the bad ones….. my nature I guess.

As I reflect back, I do have regrets on leaving veterinary practice in spite of the good memories of students at the college. Perhaps my biggest regret is not being diagnosed and treated sooner for hairy cell leukemia. This illness in retrospect certainly affected how well I functioned for over 30 years.

I am proud and at times amazed at the progress that the veterinary profession has made over the 55 years since I graduated. One of my worries is the present trend for veterinary practices to be owned and operated by large companies, utilizing hired veterinarians. This does save young veterinarians from the expense of buying or establishing a practice facility. However, being a company entity, the main goal of the corporate practices is inevitably money. I fear the loss of the "personal touch" in the corporate practices. It is very beneficial, I think, for children to have the joyful and enriching experience of having pets. Will high veterinary fees in the future mean that lower income families will not be able to afford pets or if they have pets because of cost, needed veterinary care will not be sought? In our practice and I'm sure in many private veterinary practices, we did do "freebees" or lowered our charges in special circumstances. This discretion is not there or exists in a much reduced form in the large corporate owned practices. Keith and I would never think of holidays and weekends where one or the other of us would not be available for calls. I guess we were "old school", but as more and more corporate owned practices appear, I see the trend to less and less weekend and holiday on-call service by those practices. There is already the reality of large distances between rural veterinary practices and when a number of corporate owned veterinary practices close for a weekend, the travel time required to get an emergency case to an open clinic is greatly enhanced which could be crucial for the life or death of the case. I subscribe to the thought that as veterinarians, we are a service industry.

Another troubling area for me in present day veterinary medicine is the increased demand for veterinary practices to document to minute detail procedures, surgery, and medications. Our colleagues in human medicine deal with immense amounts of "paperwork" (really done on computer) to satisfy the requirements of provincial health care, medical insurance companies, Workers' Compensation Board, etc. The shortage of medical doctors exists across North America and the non-clinical paperwork and red tape results in doctors having less time for patients or spending their evenings catching up on the "paperwork". This has led to burn-out, dissatisfaction and early retirement of doctors. Same for veterinary medicine!

In the years when I was working for the college, I did a couple locums in my summer vacation time. What astounded me was the marked increase in the "paperwork" since the time when I left private veterinary practice. Of course, accurate records are very important but I wonder if meeting the required regulations has gone too far…..to me, some of it all has just added more stress and has taken the "fun" out of veterinary practice. There are now some artificial intelligence (AI) programs designed to assist veterinary record keeping. Having no experience with them, I think that they could be of benefit but inevitably I wonder if they will add to the cost of veterinary fees. I wonder if too much "legalese" is taking over the veterinary profession?

In recent years, while waiting in a medical clinic examination room, I stared at a sign on the door that said, "No more than two questions per visit". I fervently hope that my young veterinary colleagues do not let veterinary practice regress to that level.

As I mentioned previously, the main impetus for establishing the Western College of Veterinary Medicine over 55 years ago was the shortage of veterinarians for rural areas. It is extremely perplexing that this problem still exists today in western Canada.

I don't know the answers to the problem of maintaining rural veterinary practices. Certainly graduating more veterinarians is a requirement but getting them to locate to rural areas is the complex problem. My first years in practice in the Wainwright area featured many small farms with a few milk cows, pigs, chickens and sheep. In the last 55 years these small farmers have retired or had been bought out. The Canadian beef herd has decreased; more farmland is diverted to crop production rather than livestock production. Milk processing plants have left smaller cities and amalgamated to Edmonton and Calgary; this has lead to many dairy operations in more remote areas of Alberta to discontinue operation due to the long distance to haul milk to market. Rural Alberta towns and villages lose businesses due to the big-box stores in the city; as the local businesses cease, so does the rural population. How does a dying small town have any chance of attracting a veterinarian? Fewer livestock farms and fewer residents are not very conducive to attracting or maintaining a rural veterinary practice.

In the 1970's, when Peter Lougheed was Premier of Alberta, he made attempts to revitalize rural Alberta such as building provincial buildings in rural towns and locating a number of government service agencies to smaller towns; all this at least created employment in smaller towns. I think he had the right idea, however, when the revenue from oil and gas fell and burgeoning government deficits led to successive governments consolidating government services to the cities.

We have had programs of grants and government built veterinary clinics to attract veterinarians to remote rural areas. We also have in some cases of Alberta, government subsidized payments for designated veterinary services for food producing animals. These measures are certainly of some benefit.

The World Economic Forum (WEF) is promoting the concept of "15- minute cities". I think the concept is nonsense for Calgary and Edmonton. Why not stop their further expansion over farmland? Let those two large cities revitalize their poorer run-down areas. We need to relocate industries and people to rural areas. Why not build "15- minute cities" in rural areas of the province? From my observation Edmonton and Calgary are in a hopeless situation of satisfying demand for more ring roads, subways and rapid transit. Is it time to rethink what we are doing?

I also think that people need to grow and raise more of their own food, much of which could be done in urban areas. About

THOUGHTS: FUTURE OF THE VETERINARY PROFESSION

20 to 40% of plant-based food the world produces goes to waste, there are a number of causes for this waste but long-distance transportation costs are an issue that could be addressed to some degree if the world progressed back to more locally produced and processed plant foods. Similarly, 20 to 50% of animal- based food that the world produces goes to waste. We need more efficiency to reduce waste.

Population control was a topic in my second year of university in 1964/65. Since then the world's population has more than doubled but the percentage of hungry/starving people has not doubled from the 1964 level. We just need more focus on agriculture. There has been tremendous increase in rice and wheat production since 1964. Granted drought and other crop disasters occur, however, we can make further advances in food production and food preservation. There is good technology but also bad technology when it comes to food. I worry about the manufacture of artificial foods... not natural at all.

Currently in North America the pet food industry is larger than the human baby food industry. And yes, plant and animal products are needed by the pet food industry....I'm not advocating reduction of pets, society just needs a balanced approach to the food issue.

In my experience in veterinary practice, good nutrition is of major importance in prevention of disease conditions in animals. I'm sure the same applies to human medicine and somehow in the future veterinarians and doctors have to solve many nutrition issues. I think that getting back to Mother Nature's methods should be involved in that process.

Over the course of my years in practice, I dealt with small farmer clients and I also saw the rise of large feedlots, larger dairy farms and larger hog operations (so called "factory farms" by animal rights activists and welfarists). As a generalization the small farmers demonstrated a high level of concern for their animals; invariably on a large scale operation the individual animal becomes less of a concern because of numbers. Large operations usually employ workers and the level of care of the animals depends on training as well as personal dedication. Employed workers work shifts but often there is no night shift to check the animals as there is with a family operation. I recall back to my years in practice when after the 11 pm news on television, the small farmers would go out the check their livestock. We often had midnight calls for veterinary service back in those days! Unfortunately, in a large feedlot there are no night checks and "pen-deaths" would be recorded in the morning.

I have been witness to reprehensible situations on small farm operations and I also have observed terrible situations in large operations. Once I was called out to a small dairy operation; his replacement dairy heifers were dying. The heifers were being kept in a large corral with a wooden shed for shelter. Their bellies were full…..he was feeding them hay free choice but analysis revealed that the hay was of extremely low quality (very low energy and protein levels). The weather at the time was in the -30 degree range; the heifers were eating all they could. Due to the poor quality feed, they were unable to maintain body heat and were starving to death in the cold. Some would call the owner cruel and guilty of animal abuse, but the problem was more that of lack of animal nutrition knowledge.

Animal rights people criticize the large dairy operation and bemoan the fact that the replacement dairy heifers are kept confined in a small pen in a barn. Cruel, they say in terms of limited space but they are ignorant to the fact that there are temperature and humidity controls in the dairy barn and the fact that the feed ration has been formulated by a nutritional specialist.

I have witnessed the situation at a large feedlot that had just purchased a hydraulic cattle squeeze for processing the feedlot

THOUGHTS: FUTURE OF THE VETERINARY PROFESSION

cattle. Either out of cruelty or again ignorance, the feedlot worker was using the tailgate as a battering ram against the hind quarters of the cattle to get the cattle to step forward. Hydraulics used excessively created a lot of pressure and severe bruising injuries.

I guess I'm trying to say that things are not either totally black or white. Yes knowingly or unknowingly some things are not ideal on the large livestock operations but I subscribe to the approach of striving to make improvements rather than elimination of the large animal operations.

The large so called "factory farms" have evolved partly due to the fact that the profit per animal unit is very low so large numbers are essential to maintaining a viable operation. People forget that in reality we do have cheap food in North America, perhaps if we had paid more for eggs and meat smaller farm operations would have been viable and we would not have had the evolution of the factory farms? In North America, the % of personal income spent on food is low compared to many other countries of the world, however, are our priorities cell phones, expensive homes, expensive cars, etc. over food? The issue is complex when one thinks about it.

More than once I have had these questions posed to me: (1) Aren't you a bit of a hypocrite to work with food producing animals when you know that they will be cruelly slaughtered? (2) Don't you feel like a hypocrite raising your own animals for slaughter?

I admit that I have had those thoughts myself. Times like when I'm out in the pasture and cow 11C hurries over to give a jealous head bunt to scare off cow 6C that I am scratching on the back. My rationale is that mankind has kept animals for food purposes for centuries. If livestock production is carried out, I think the onus is to afford the animals humane life free from hunger and pain. When one thinks seriously, Mother Nature can be cruel….

there are times when wild animals starve to death because of drought, flooding or excessive snow cover. A cat playing with a mouse cannot be regarded as humane for the mouse.

Yes, there is a nastiness to a slaughterhouse, but all living creatures have to die at some point. In Canada we do have government regulations to make methods of killing animals more humane. I admit they are hard to perceive as humane but compare it to a deer being slowly chewed to death by a pack of wolves. And yes, there are times when the kill process for an animal does not go well because of human carelessness or fatigue of the worker. I worked in slaughterhouses as a veterinary student and overall methods of kill since then have improved: example of shooting a bull in the head with a rifle (missing the correct area of the head) versus a bolt stun gun which is placed close to the head, resulting in a more certain stun.

I confess, I do own a rifle and a shotgun and have owned a number of other guns. Yes, I have hunted deer, grouse and ducks for meat to eat. Again, there are those who would say that it is hypocritical for a veterinarian to hunt. I do have some appreciation for their views, I guess my justification for owning guns also relates to the fact that there are bears and cougars in the area where we have lived and having protection is an issue. As a cattle owner, I have also had a couple occasions where euthanasia of a couple of cows was required, having a rifle was a valuable necessity. From time to time, in a rural setting, guns are also required for pest control. Hypocrite or not, I guess I do have reasons for gun ownership.

Looking back, a career as a rural veterinarian can be very demanding, stressful, and also difficult for the veterinarian's wife and family. In the western provinces the mainstay of most rural practices is beef cattle and the majority of beef cattle work occurs in spring and fall. A level of other veterinary work with companion animals, sheep, swine, dairy cattle and horses is required to keep the doors of a rural practice open. Again, there is a need to revitalize rural Canada, not just for the good of the rural veterinary practice but also for the good of society.

A very real struggle for a rural veterinarian is that of trying to keep pace with advances in companion animal, equine, ovine, porcine and bovine surgery and medicine etc. I remember the many occasions attending a veterinary conference where I was often conflicted over which animal species seminar to attend.

Another reality for rural veterinary practice is that of presenting a certain appearance and demeanor for a cattle rancher and minutes later another for a small animal client. I recall finishing work on a cow, then stripping off my coveralls and rushing to the front of the clinic to attend to attend to Mrs. Jones's sick dog. I was blissfully unaware that I had a little lump of cow manure stuck on the top of my nose!

In reflection, I sometimes think my career as a rural veterinarian involved being "a little bit of everything, but not a lot of anything." Thankfully, for today's rural veterinarians there are now many specialized veterinary practices to enable referral of difficult or complex cases. For many of my practice years, there was not the availability of endoscopes, ultrasound, digital radiography, in-clinic blood analyzers etc.

My career as a rural veterinarian was a learning curve but I think that is true for most of society.

Given the importance that companion animals have in today's society, I think that the future of small animal veterinarians is assured. I caution them to remember to find ways to address after-hour and holiday service to maintain a positive perception by the public.

When the era of the motor vehicle began, the number of horses decreased markedly. Veterinary colleges started to relegate equine medicine and surgery to minor roles in veterinary curriculum. Today the horse has become popular for recreation, companionship and sport. I foresee a strong demand for equine veterinarians.

The "animal food" industries (beef, dairy, hogs, sheep and poultry) are being assaulted by various animal rights/wellfarist groups, vegan only groups, technocrats producing "man-made" foods and radical climate change activists. I fervently hope that common sense will come to be in a middle ground for those industries. The challenge for food animal veterinarians will be to educate the public and promote reasonable public perception in regards to food animal production.

Over the last 55 years there has been a virtual explosion in veterinary medical knowledge, surgery and technology. A big debate in whether veterinary colleges should institute specialization training of veterinary undergraduates versus the traditional general training.

I worry about the future for rural veterinary practitioners. It does take a special type of personality for a veterinarian (and their spouse as well) to adapt to life and career in smaller communities. The challenges of rural veterinary practice are many; the reward is not only helping the animals but also the opportunity to find friendships with "salt of the earth people" (our farmers and ranchers).

When I reflect back on the friendships and hospitality of the animal owners, students and ex-coworkers over my career as a rural veterinarian; I do feel very rewarded!

References

1. Vitamin A deficiency in beef calves
   https://vetmed.iastate.edu>V...

2. Bladder stones (obstructive urolithiasis) in cattle
   https://industry.nt.gov.au>... (PDF)

3. Bovine Viral Diarrhea: Background, Management and Control
   https://www.vet.cornell.edu>nyschap

4. Coccidiosis In Cattle
   http://open.alberta.ca>publications

5. Coccidiosis in Cattle – Merck Veterinary Manual
   https://www.merckvetmanual.com>

6. Grain poisoning of cattle and sheep
   https://www.dpi.nsw.gov.au>... [PDF]

7. Bovine Enteric Colibacillosis – ScienceDirect.com
   https://www.sciencedirect.com> pdf

8. Tetanus in Horses – Merck Veterinary Manual
   https://www.merckvetmanual.com>...

9. Clinical Features, Diagnosis and Treatment of Western Equine Encephalitis
   https://www.cdc.gov>wee>hcp

10. Canine Distemper
    https://www.avma.org>petcare

11. Government of Alberta
    http://open.alberta.ca>publications
    Veterinary Profession Act – Open Government Program

12. Mayo Clinic
    https://www.mayoclinic.org>syc-...
    Hairy Cell Leukemia – Symptoms and Causes

13. Wikipedia
    http://en.wikipedia.org>wiki>R...
    Rabies is a viral disease that causes encephalitis in humans and other mammals

14. National Institutes of Health (NIH)(gov)
    www.ncbi.nim.nih.gov
    Conserving wildlife in a changing world: understanding capture myopathy

15. The Musk Oxen of Gango: Borealis Book Publishers
    http://www.borealispress.com>rid

16. Canine parvovirus
    https://www.avma.org>petcare

17. Warble Control in Alberta
    https://open.alberta.ca>do [PDF]

18. Brucellosis in Cattle
    https://www.merckvetmanual.com>....

19. Bovine Tuberculosis – Fact Sheet
    https://inspection.canada.ca>fact-...

20. Bovine Spongiform Encephalopathy (BSE)
    Centers for Disease Control and Prevention
    https://www.cdc.gov

Printed in Canada